Glass House Books

No Middle Name

Tilly Brasch spent her early years in the north and west of Queensland. After marriage to Kevin, she moved to Brisbane and raised two children, Jacoba and Riley.

When the children were in their teens, Tilly embarked on an administrative career in tertiary education. During this time, she gained an Arts degree and discovered the joy of writing.

After the onset of Riley's mental illness, Tilly lobbied politicians and appeared in the media in an effort to expose the plight of these neglected members of our community. This book, No Middle Name, is an extension of her desire to raise public awareness, reform the health system, and improve the quality of life for those who still suffer as Riley did.

Tilly's interests include keeping fit, and a love of words, both in the reading and writing context. She is avidly committed to solving every crossword she encounters. Her passion is for her two granddaughters, Madison and Darcy.

Glass House Books
Brisbane

GHB

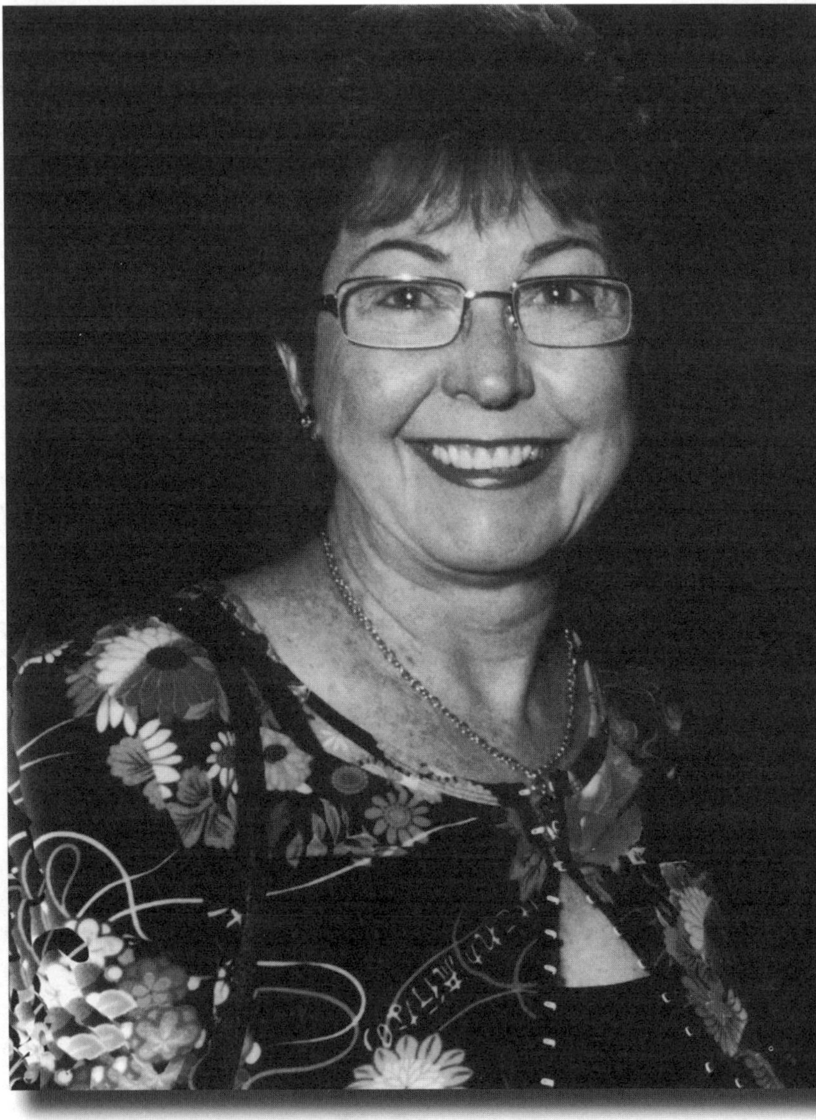

No Middle Name

Tilly Brasch

Glass House Books
Brisbane

GHB

***G**lass **H**ouse **B**ooks*
an imprint of Interactive Publications
Treetop Studio • 9 Kuhler Court
Carindale, Queensland, Australia 4152
sales@ipoz.biz
www.ipoz.biz/ghb/ghb.htm

First published by Glass House Books, 2005

Printed in 18 pt Century Schoolbook Bold on 11 pt Century Schoolbook by Harding Colour and Watson and Ferguson, Queensland, Australia. Made, printed and bound in Australia.

National Library of Australia
Cataloguing-in-Publication data:

Brasch, Tilly.
No middle name.

Bibliography.
Includes index.
ISBN 1 876819 90 1.

1. Brasch, Riley. 2. Mentally ill - Queensland - Biography.
3. Mentally ill - Family relationships. I. Title.

616.890092

for Madison and Darcy to whom I entrust these precious memories.

Acknowledgments

When I think of acknowledgements, my first thought goes to my sister, Narelle. Her unstinting belief in my ability to write Riley's story, as well as the necessity to tell his story, became my motivation.

Lauren Elise Daniels is a new friend, but one that I feel I was always destined to meet. Lauren's expertise with the written word, her empathy, and understanding of the emotional difficulties that often impeded my writing efforts, gave me the ability and courage to develop my first draft to a manuscript worthy of sending off to a publisher. Lauren also led a writing group that had a significant impact on my confidence to continue with Riley's story: Julie Graffe, Erica Hart, Madonna Perkins, and Rae Peters– all talented writers who gave me the benefit of their writing skills.

For twenty years, Mark Burton's artistry with the written word became the standard to which I aspired. And Mark's meticulous literary eye put polish on my final draft.

During the writing of Riley's story, an isolating and solitary process, my husband Kevin patiently indulged me in my obsessive commitment to sit at the computer in a world of my own. He gave me all the space that I needed to write Riley's story.

'Thank you' is inadequate to express what I wish to say to my daughter, Jacoba. Coby has given me the joy of being a grandmother. The births of Madison and Darcy marked my emotional rebirth after Riley's death. Now, my every day is brimful with the delight of boisterous, laughing children. Madi and Darcy heap my heart full with happiness.

I am grateful to my publisher, Dr David Reiter, for the opportunity to put Riley's story before the public. My appreciation of David's gentle guidance and his confidence in my ability to develop No Middle Name to a standard that fills me with pride, has grown steadily throughout the editing process. I also thank Assistant Editor Anne Marshall, who has edited my work in a supportive manner.

But, most of all, thank you to Riley whose short life enriched mine in so many wonderful ways. I am a better person for having been his mother.

Contents

Prologue

Seventeenth Century playwright, Pierre Cornielle, wrote that "Telling one's sorrows often brings comfort". I knew from the earliest days after we lost Riley that eventually I would *tell* his life story. The compulsion to do so was always there, but the courage was not. More than seven years have passed and it is only now that I can find that courage to confront the past in such a deliberate manner.

Indeed, I have found great comfort in gathering together all the elements of Riley's life and reviving memories of him through my words. But I have had my difficult moments along the way.

The emotional demand of writing Riley's story has not been my only dilemma. I have wrestled with my conscience from the start, asking "Am I revealing too much of Riley's life? Am I exposing him to the world? Would he approve?"

But I can hear him saying, "Go for it, Mum. Tell them how it was. There are others like me out there, and they need to know. You can do it."

I have been open and honest in telling it how it was. Some of the things I have revealed have caused me great anxiety. Do I need to be this brutally honest? Could I leave some things out, and fudge a little with the truth? No, I couldn't. Only the truth will do justice to Riley's memory. But I think that I have shown him to be a likeable young man, neither a saint nor a sinner.

My first draft of Riley's story was full of anger and rage, but in subsequent drafts, I have been able to move on from those negative emotions. To simply put my anger into words has been a healing process and I can now let them go.

Of course, I have had to delve into my memories to write about Riley's life. Some of my memories are clear, but others have only come to me in fragments, as if my mind and heart are reluctant to let them go. However, once I began to exhume these memories from the deepest parts of my mind, so many more emerged.

Through the process of writing this story as an exposition of Riley's twenty-six years, a wonderful and unexpected thing happened. My words became a revelation, as if I was reading an unknown story and, only page by page, was the content being made known to me, revealing a person that I was not aware of when he was alive: although my love for Riley can never be in doubt, I realize that I also *like* him! Previously, we shared a conglomeration of disjointed bits and pieces where the difficulties and miseries were foremost in my memory. But now I can see that we often had fun and laughed easily with each other. Now I am conscious of the companionship that we shared and this gives me comfort.

This confirms yet another reason that I had for writing Riley's story. Not many people knew the 'real' Riley — the caring, courageous, funny lad. In general, because of his illness, prejudicial assumptions were made about him and I was not comfortable with this. I had to resist being constantly defensive on his behalf. Silence became my method of coping. But I can no longer be silent. I hope that, by reading this story, you will see my son as a whole person, not just one who was 'mentally ill'. He didn't want to be mentally ill. He couldn't help being it. I want you to understand that part of him that wasn't affected by his illness.

A dear friend and mentor wrote after reading the first draft of Riley's story:

"Your writing shows that some parts of his life were not disasters. This ability to trust in such a rough world led him to disaster, but there is something pure about that trust, so pure that most of us lose it."

I have come to see this pure quality in my son through reading my own story. But it is Riley's life and how he lived that life that is pure, not my writing.

"Did I do good, Riley?" I would ask.

"Yes, Mum, you done good," he would assure me.

Although Riley had, and still has, a loving father and sister, this is my story about him. I do not presume to speak for Kevin or Jacoba (Coby), nor does my exclusion of them imply that I alone shared in Riley's life and fought the battle with, and for, him. We are a tight-knit family and Riley will continue to be held lovingly in our hearts. We all tried to the point of emotional and physical exhaustion to give Riley a meaningful life, to affect changes both for him and within our community. We failed, but this is not a story about failure – this is my story about my son.

I have changed the names of everyone involved except my immediate family, and the words of public figures I quote are already in the public domain. I have also changed the names of schools, hospitals, and accommodation to prevent identification and embarrassment. I do not intend to apportion blame or to censure anyone. Sometimes though, the truth exposes flaws in our attitudes and social structure, which makes us uncomfortable but which can lead to necessary changes.

Above all, the context and essence of all events are faithfully represented.

Read my words with your eyes, but understand them with your heart. Not just for Riley, but for those who are like Riley and still battling unbeatable odds.

Chapter 1

For almost twenty-six years, I had a son whose flesh I could touch and smell, whose jokes made me laugh, whose kindness and tolerance made me proud. Riley's daily life and emotions were entwined with mine. He shaped my life.

But while I slept, my son died.

Now all I have are memories that I cannot hold in my arms. And Riley will not share the future with me. Even so, Riley still affects my life in countless ways. Some memories still make me laugh, but most make me sad.

In 1971, the year of Riley's birth, Brisbane pulsated in opposition to the State of Emergency declared by Queensland's Bjelke-Petersen government, which had denied the democratic rights of citizens to protest, and in particular against the forthcoming Springbok rugby tour which embodied the racist principles of apartheid. But my husband Kevin and I were more concerned about the impending birth of our second child.

Prior to Riley's birth, in the fifth month of my pregnancy, I expressed concern to my obstetrician that I seemed to be very small. "Some people don't realise that I'm pregnant. Shouldn't I be bigger than this?" I asked.

Dr Fry was a weary man of few words and did not indulge in friendly chatter. During appointments, matters pertaining to my pregnancy were dealt with efficiently and quickly. A personal rapport was never established. "The baby will grow rapidly during this second trimester. We'll see how things are going at your next appointment," he responded.

At the next appointment, my size had not increased much, but I was assured that rapid growth would occur during the last trimester. Dr Fry had no doubt that I "would get a spurt on". But six weeks before the expected birth date, he confirmed that the baby's head was smaller than it should be, so I began weekly oestrogen tests, which monitored the baby's progress.

"Every detail about the baby's development, except its sex, can be interpreted from these tests," he assured me. This was the zenith of medical technology in 1971, before the advent of amniocentesis and ultrasounds. "If the tests reveal a problem, I'll do an emergency caesarean delivery. But unless there are indications to the contrary, the baby is better off in the womb, rather than taking its chances outside in a humidicrib."

However, Riley came naturally fourteen days after the expected date of arrival. It was a quick and easy birth.

He was born on a mild winter's day, two weeks past his due date, on 15 July 1971, at 11.35am. I always told Riley that he was born just in time for lunch. We also told him, tongue-in-cheek, that he didn't have a middle name because we couldn't afford one, but in later years when he was at kindergarten I overheard the roll call one day for Riley John Brasch.

"Riley hasn't got a middle name," I protested to the director, "John is not part of his name."

"I know," she replied, "but he decided that he wanted to be Riley John Brasch because all the other children have middle names, and he wants one too."

I paused. "Well, if he wants to be Riley John Brasch, then let him be." We didn't formalise this name change and Riley often joked about it in later life, telling us that he was a deprived child, a child without a middle name. We had purposely avoided giving our children middle names because they often become a source of embarrassment in later life, but Riley decided differently. "Deciding his own decides" as he later expressed himself, became a hallmark of Riley's character as he grew up.

Riley was described to me as a 'frail' baby, weighing 5 lb 12 oz (2608 g). Dr Fry explained that the baby was dysmature because of placental insufficiency. Dysmaturity, or intrauterine growth retardation, describes an infant of significantly low birth weight, who is born postmature (later than forty-two weeks) rather than premature. This is caused by a failure of the placenta to supply adequate oxygen and nutrition to the foetus during gestation.

When all medical procedures had been completed after the

birth, while I was still drifting in the hazy world of medication and post-birth euphoria, I watched the doctor examine the placenta in a bucket, beside the delivery table.

"Look at this. All this black stuff. Dead. Fair bit of it's dead. I'd say seventy per cent of it is dead. This little fellow has been starved of oxygen and nutrition during the pregnancy. What's his name?" the doctor asked. Lack of oxygen would have explained the distinct blue colour of his skin that I remember being aware of when Riley was delivered.

"Riley," I replied. Saying his name for the first time sealed the bond that nature intended. I was besotted with instantaneous maternal love.

"Sounds like you should be driving him, not giving birth to him." The doctor was referring to the classic Riley sports car. And, although I was concerned about the outcome of the placental examination, I was not alert enough to ask probing questions.

"Is he alright? He'll be alright, won't he?" was the best I could manage.

"He's frail and smaller than we'd like," the doctor explained. "We'll keep him here for a while and see that he gets off to a good start. Stabilise him. But don't you worry. He'll catch up before you know what's what."

I should have expected more information from the doctor, but I had a simple trust that the medical profession would support us through whatever health issues the future might hold.

"You'll be fine, little man," I whispered in my baby's tiny, tissue-like ear before he was whisked away from me. "We'll be okay."

Riley remained in the frail nursery of the maternity hospital to receive special care for two weeks after I was discharged. I had a two-year-old daughter at home, Coby, who also needed mothering. Walking away from the hospital without my baby in my arms was the hardest thing that I had done at that point in my life and it filled me with despair. I felt empty, bereft of sensation. 'How do young women who give their babies up for adoption do this?' I pondered. 'How can they just walk away? I think I would die from a broken heart.' I empathised with all those mothers who had made such a heart-wrenching departure. At least I could come back for my little one.

The woman who had roomed with me left hospital at the same time as I did, but with her baby cradled in her arms. I lingered at a distance down the corridor so that I didn't have to confront them. But I could see her from the corner of my eye, cuddling her baby, bubbling with joy. I felt miserable.

In the following days, Kevin kept assuring me that it was better for Riley to remain in hospital, receiving the care that I was not able to give him at home. "Don't upset yourself," he pleaded. "He'll be fine, you'll see. We'll have him home in no time."

To ease my wretchedness in the following fortnight, my parents took me to the hospital daily to spend time with Riley.

Initially, because of his fragile health, I was not allowed to hold Riley. I could only look at him through a glass window, a tragic foreshadowing of what would happen later in Riley's life. Still, I had no difficulty identifying my baby from all the other little ones. At first, they all looked the same: tiny, frail, swathed in bunny-rugs with just their little heads peeking through, but one looked like a wizened little chimpanzee with Prince Charles ears. This one was mine. Even though we were separated by glass, my nose filled with the smell of his baby-soft skin.

I was not permitted to breast-feed Riley, and was given tablets to dry my milk. I couldn't even express my milk for Riley's bottle-feeds. I was naive and felt intimidated by the authority of the nursing staff.

After a few days, I was allowed to hold Riley briefly once a day, and eventually my visits included feeding him one bottle daily, with the remainder of his bottles being held to his mouth as he lay in his crib — cot feeding, they called it. Feeding Riley proved to be challenging because he held his tongue against the roof of his mouth, making it difficult to get the teat into the correct position for him to suck.

I asked the big, robust religious sister in charge of the frail nursery, "How can I get this teat in? It keeps going under his tongue."

"Like this," she replied as she pinched his tiny toes. "When he's screaming, he will drop his tongue to draw breath, and that's when you pop the teat in."

I was bewildered, and never resorted to this tactic. I preferred patience and persistence.

And his bath, every second day, consisted of a quick wipe-over with a damp cloth. There were precious few opportunities to cuddle this tiny baby as medical advice continued to keep me at a physical distance from my son. "Too much handling will harm him. We must avoid any non-essential contact." The inclusive 'we' drew me into impersonal nursing procedures.

Twenty-nine years later when my first granddaughter was born sixteen weeks premature, weighing 790g, or 1lb 12oz, Kangaroo Cuddling, a very intimate form of mother-child physical contact in which the tiny infant is removed from its humidicrib and placed between the mother's breasts, skin to skin, was encouraged from her earliest days. This closeness promotes physical development and well-being in the delicate infant and significantly contributes to survival. Times change.

But nature works in wondrous ways. Although I had not lactated for three weeks, my maternal instinct was so strong that when the hospital phoned to tell me I could bring my baby home, I immediately began to produce copious amounts of milk. On arrival at the hospital a short time later, I was euphoric and announced: "I have enough milk to feed quads! It's a miracle! I can breast-feed my baby!"

I was met with an emphatic 'no'. "It will be too difficult for you because of his tongue, and you'll only stress the baby. You'll have to take those tablets again to dry your milk."

Not me, I thought, I'm not taking any more tablets. Despite the discomfort of engorgement because I wasn't breast-feeding Riley, I let my milk dry out naturally. Lactation completed nature's birth cycle and it was physical proof of the strong bond that I had with my son in spite of the medical barriers that had marked the first three weeks of our relationship.

Following Riley's release from hospital, his health continued to be monitored by a Child Welfare nurse who visited our home every second day for several weeks. Not handling him continued to be a priority and she always weighed him in his bassinet, in his clothes. The normal procedure is to weigh just a naked, or near naked baby.

"Remember now. Only pick him up for every second feed, and baths every other day. He mustn't be handled any more than is absolutely necessary. And no visitors! Visitors always want to pick the baby up. They'll be a problem. And they might bring germs too. You have to be tough for the baby's sake."

What could I do? I longed to hold and cuddle my baby, but a fear had been instilled into me that physical contact would harm him.

But in time, Riley did reach the point where I could treat him as a normal baby. He was a delightful little person, whom I often remarked must have read the book on how to be a good and cooperative baby. Unlike Coby, whose incessant crying with colic demanded my attention for most of the day and night for many long months, Riley slept so well and so long, I would stand by his bassinet willing him to wake up so that I could hold him and breathe in his baby smell and feel his baby-soft skin.

Apart from the delivery room revelations about the placenta, I was given no further information, nor was any long-term prognosis made about how dysmaturity and placental insufficiency might affect Riley's physical and mental development. Explanations were not given and questions were not asked. I know now that I should have asked questions and demanded answers, but I had a background where respect for the medical profession precluded patient interrogation. That was how it happened in the early 1970s. Two follow-up appointments with a paediatrician during Riley's first year did not indicate any cause for concern. The prognosis at each visit was that he was 'doing nicely, just a little on the small side.'

But, with hindsight, I can confess to always having a niggling concern about the circumstances of his birth, and how this might impact on him in later life. I was constantly watchful, always looking for reassurance that Riley was developing normally. Or was he?

Chapter 2

In the few seconds that it took me to run to Riley's rescue, I saw the older, stronger boy push Riley's head under the water again. As Riley's face broke the surface of the wading pool, he smiled at his tormentor.

I clutched him to me. "Why did you let him do that?" I implored. "Why did you smile at him? He was being unkind to you."

"No, he's nice Mummy. He's my new friend. He's playing with me." Riley was four years old. I didn't know it then, but this was to be a potent prophecy of how Riley experienced relationships throughout his life.

In the same year, I took Coby to a local paediatrician because of recurring bronchitis. Dr Newton was popular with other young mothers in my circle of friends. He was a big grandfatherly man with steel grey hair, and although he had a fearsome reputation for being impatient with mothers whom he considered were foolish, he was respected for his dedication and brilliance as a practitioner.

I soon learned that although Dr Newton was a paediatrician, he was like the family doctor of an earlier era. He kept an eye on all the family. "You're looking a bit thin, Mother. Children a bit demanding? You've got to take time for yourself, you know."

Riley was always a well-behaved little boy and stood patiently at my knee while Coby was examined. However, even before Dr Newton broached the subject, I saw by his frequent glances at Riley that he was more interested in my son than my daughter.

"Do you mind if I have a look at your little fellow? He seems quite small. How old is he? Tell me about him." I told the doctor all that I knew of Riley's medical history, and after examining Riley, he advised, "I'm going to set up some appointments for Riley at a hospital that has the specialists and resources to do a thorough battery of tests. First of all, they'll determine that there are no undiagnosed reasons for his size, and, if all is well there, they will do a bone age test. By x-raying Riley's wrist, the doctors will be able to compare him with other children of the same age to determine his relative maturity, and they will also be able to estimate his height as an adult. It might be that growth hormones will benefit him later on. But let's hand it all over to the specialists, shall we?"

With Dr Newton's letter of referral in hand, we began an annual pilgrimage to the children's hospital where another paediatrician and an endocrinologist monitored Riley's progress for the next five or six years. However, when all the tests and measurements were completed each year, Riley's physical development was always better than the criteria required to be treated with hormones.

At each of these visits, I asked questions about his mental development in relation to his birth, and in particular, I sought reassurance from all of the doctors treating Riley about some of the behavioural quirks that were concerning me.

"Now, Mother," Dr Newton began, placing his hand gently on my shoulder, "we've been through all this before. You are worrying needlessly. But then, mothers do worry, don't they? I should know. I see enough of them. Riley's only problem is that he is small. You are small. Your husband is not a big man. So Riley will most likely always be small. Perhaps he will become a jockey. Most jockeys were dysmature at birth. Did you know that? And Prime Minister Billy McMahon. Small, with those big flappy ears like Riley's. He was most likely dysmature. Nothing wrong with him, is there? Riley will be fine. You'll see. Give him time."

In the early years of Riley's life, I was familiar with this response to my constant queries about the circumstances of his birth and possible repercussions. The doctors that we consulted as he was growing up all dismissed any connection between Riley's birth and his mental development. But I could never shake off my doubts and I continued to feel uneasy about his birth and how he was developing intellectually.

When he was a little fellow, I could put him in a strange cot when we were out visiting, and he would go to sleep without fussing. Most toddlers would object to a strange bed. I remember watching him once, out of sight, when I put him into a friend's cot. He just had a look around, lay down, and went to sleep.

The placid nature that had been endearing to me when he was an infant now unsettled me. He seemed content in his own world and as he grew older, he didn't seem to 'connect' with other children. He was timid and vulnerable, yet he was unruffled by strange faces, strange places, and strange events. His reaction to life was benign.

It was during these annual medical tests that I became increasingly aware of Riley's reaction to pain. His appointments required him to have repetitive blood tests, but he never cried. He withstood whatever they did to him without a flinch. At first I thought he was a brave little boy, but as time passed, I became conscious of a consistent pattern of stoicism. I was distressed, not so much at having to present my child for painful medical procedures, but at his unusual fortitude. Other children would have had to be physically restrained, screaming and kicking, but not Riley.

I have a vivid memory of myself pleading with him to cry. "Please cry, Riley. It's okay to cry. That's what other little children do. Please cry, son." But he didn't. He never did. I have tried to remember a time when I might have comforted Riley because pain had made him cry, but I cannot. Perhaps even then, when he was only a little boy, he was experiencing pain differently to others.

Etched in my memory are other occasions during Riley's childhood when he did not react to pain in a normal manner. He broke one of his front teeth in half in a school playground mishap when he was seven. The pain must have been intense. But when I went to the school to collect him to take him to the dentist, he didn't murmur. Nor was there any protest of pain when the tooth was being fixed in the dental surgery. And he fell off a horse when he was eleven years old and broke his arm. But he didn't cry. It was the twisted arm and the distinct crack that I heard that alerted me to the fracture, not his tears. At no stage while being transported to hospital or while his arm was being attended to did he cry.

From memories that I have of discussing pain and a normal reaction to pain with him later in his life, I know that Riley thought pain was his due, what he was worthy of. He expected the world to punish and hurt him. Perhaps even then, when he was little, these annual episodes with the specialists were signs of what the future held for him and his family.

Our willingness to accept medical assurances about the circumstances of Riley's birth in 1971, as well as the failure of the medical profession to act on my concerns in subsequent years, would not happen now. It is now common for people to take recourse at law and aggressively seek answers to health matters that they believe are caused by oversight or medical negligence. From the earliest days of Riley's life, even before he was born, I intuitively felt that something was amiss, but my disquiet was so consistently dismissed or ignored by those from whom I sought help, I became full of self-doubt and wondered if the only problem was with me. Was I unnecessarily overanxious and overprotective of my son?

Nonetheless, my maternal instincts told me that I had cause to be concerned despite the learned opinions of medical experts. The medical profession has an entrenched history of closing ranks, where protection of self, one's colleagues, and the profession's reputation takes priority over admissions of error or fallibility. I am in no doubt that Riley was failed in many ways, first by nature and then by the human elements that came into his life.

My concerns that things were not right for Riley increased as he got older. He was an appealing toddler with blond curly hair framing his elfin face, but as he got to the stage of interacting with other children, it was increasingly apparent to me that his demeanour was different. The differences that I was aware of were niggly little mannerisms that I found hard to explain to others and it usually felt silly when I tried to put them into words. He always seemed to be on the edge of a group, not knowing how to participate in the activity. And although it's natural that many people are not leaders, Riley was not even a follower. He just seemed to be there, in whatever surroundings we placed him, without understanding why he was there or what was required of him. There was a palpable helplessness about Riley and I feared for him when he was out of my sight and beyond my protection.

But there were some moments that did give us heart during Riley's early years. "Go go go! You're nearly there, Riley. A few more strokes. You can do it! One more stroke! Yeah! You've done it!" Riley had just completed swimming his first length of a twenty-five-metre pool. He was five.

Because Kevin and I were aware, even at this early stage, of Riley's awkwardness with group activities, we tried to create opportunities for him to participate in activities as an individual, with some success.

Starting in Grade One, Riley successfully took part in a swimming club that had a graded handicap system that made all swimmers equally competitive. Each individual swimmer was handicapped according to his or her own best time, rather than the 'scratch' system where all swimmers dive from the blocks on the starter's gun, as they do in the Olympics. This system gave even the weakest swimmer the opportunity to beat the strongest if the handicapping was calculated accurately. Riley won many trophies and enjoyed the camps that the swimming club conducted for its young members. He had many friends and interacted well with the adult officials. Swimming club was a happy place for Riley. But Kevin and I were never far away.

In games with neighbourhood children, Riley was always the one who never caught the others in a game of 'Chase' but was always caught when he was chased. And he never found anyone when they played 'Hide-and-Seek' but was always the first found when he hid. When they rode off on their bikes, he was always last and alone, trying to catch up.

Another group of boys in our neighbourhood terrorised him when I sent him to our local convenience store.

"Please don't make me to go to the shop, Mum. I'm scared of those boys on the corner." His pleas to be spared from the unkindness of these boys still ring in my ears. I soon learned not to ask him to do this chore.

For the same reason, Riley would not catch the bus from the stop outside the shop. He begged us not to interfere by confronting the boys or their parents because he knew, and we had to agree, that doing so would only worsen matters. But the bullying behaviour of these boys not only took away some of Riley's liberty to be carefree in his own neighbourhood, it also undermined what little confidence he did have, making him more timid and uncertain of his place with his peers.

We were always aware of Riley's low self esteem and bolstered him at every opportunity by praising him and highlighting his hard-won achievements, yet our praise counted for nothing when we overheard other boys taunting him that he was a *retard, a loser, a drop-kick, pizza face* and other words which are not in our vocabulary.

But there were times when Riley's confidence soared. Through Kevin's involvement in Rugby League, Riley became a ball boy and ran the sideline for many important games, including State of Origin, grand finals, and international tests. All the prominent players knew Riley because of Kevin, and he was delighted when heroes of the game took the time to chat to him or scruffle his hair. After a game, his chest puffed out as he recounted taking sand out to the goal kicker. "Mal said, 'Thanks, young Braschie', Mum. He knows me!" He was thrilled.

However, if Riley made the early discovery that his social world was not always kind, school quickly became the next painful period in his life. Apart from his inability to interact easily with his peers, the processes of learning were consistently elusive. At each level of his education, we hoped that the key would be found to unlock the door to knowledge. With each new teacher we hoped that things would fall into place for him. Surely there was a teacher who could connect with him and unravel his bewilderment.

But school was always a place of mystery for Riley. He didn't bring home notes, messages, or homework, and it wasn't because he was lazy or rebellious. He just didn't seem to understand the daily procedures. He had no awareness of routine, and therefore never established nor followed one. This never altered throughout his life. Nor did he ever object to what must have been a frightening and overwhelming environment for him: there were never any tantrums about going to school even though he must have been miserable there.

When he was in Grade Three, his teacher took me aside. "Mrs Brasch, I'm worried about Riley's maths. He just doesn't seem to be grasping the basic concepts. For some time now, I've been trying to work with him one-on-one, and today, we spent a whole lesson together. Just Riley and me. I thought I was making progress, because he watched and listened so intently. I really thought he was taking it all in. But when I asked him if he understood, he looked at me and said, 'Miss Grant. You're very beautiful. Especially your eyes'." Clearly frustrated, she was uncertain how to offer Riley the academic basics he required. Like us, she was stumped.

Kevin and I worked diligently on schoolwork with Riley at home, but the results mostly reflected our efforts, not his. Many times, because he didn't bring home correct information, I helped him with homework from page ten, exercise six instead of page six, exercise ten. I remember being shattered that he was given no credit or encouragement for at least getting what he had done correct. Instead, his work was marked zero. He used to say to me, "I'm just a zero, Mum." He was always in the remedial group and he repeated one year.

We constantly tried to overcome his inability to follow a daily routine by taking him step-by-step through the sequence of events, or at least to get his thought processes going from A to B to C. But Riley's brain didn't function this logically. His defective logic was like someone who randomly flicks through the pages of a large book written in a foreign language, jumping from page 5 to 97, back to 24, then upside down and backwards, and then back to a blank page, then reading only one paragraph from every other page, and so on. The resulting story of course doesn't make sense, but this was the way *his* thought processes worked – to quote Cyndi Lauper's song 'Time after Time', his 'drum beats out of time'.

I regularly did tuck-shop duty, and observed Riley at recess time, on his own, wandering around as if he was lost, with his finger on his top lip. He had a habit of holding his chin with four of his fingers and gently touching his top lip with his index finger. He always did this when he seemed to be taking comfort within himself, as if he was withdrawing from what was happening around him. With the knowledge that I have now, I have no doubt that he was emotionally lost.

When Riley was in the early years of primary school, he was invited to other children's parties, but as he got older, the invitations ceased. His exclusion from his classmates' social network throughout his school years set him apart as a loner. Mother Teresa said "loneliness and the feeling of being unwanted is the most terrible poverty". Riley lived constantly with the poverty of loneliness.

But school did provide Riley with the opportunity to experiment with music. Much to the detriment of our poor ears, and in a test of the neighbours' tolerance, Riley attempted to master many musical instruments through school music programs. If an instrument could be transported, he brought it home. We endured mournful practice sessions on the trumpet, clarinet, saxophone, oboe, guitar, and violin.

"I hope there are no moose in the neighbourhood, Riley."

"Why, Mum?"

"That sounds like a moose mating call to me."

He did, however, gain Honours for his first piano exam. He also achieved similar grades for Speech and Drama.

From an early age, Riley had a high standard of verbal expression, which reflected not only his Speech and Drama training, but also the every day usage of vocabulary in our home. This often misled people to think that Riley had intellectual abilities that, in fact, he didn't. His excellent verbal skills didn't follow through to competent actions.

When the children were little, we had a rule that when we travelled in the car as a family, we never played the radio or tape deck. This was a time for communication and word games. A favourite was the shopping list game:

"I went to the shop and I bought an apple."

"I went to the shop and I bought an apple and some eggs." The following item had to start with the last letter of the previous item.

"I went to the shop and I bought an apple, some eggs, and sugar." And so on.

We also played a car number plate game, which required a sentence to be made up from the three letters of the plate: AVV991 – Anthony Voted Vigorously. Or CEJ451 – Colin Exited Jumping.

Of course, 'I Spy' was one of many other games that occupied our driving time. One of Riley's favourite clues started with 'N'. The answer? 'Nure (manure). "Gotcha that time," he gloated victoriously, thinking he had caught us out with one that he used every time we played the game.

We also enjoyed thinking of songs that had a particular theme, perhaps titles that contained a colour, or titles that included a girl's name. Songs like 'I Dream of Jeanie with the Light Brown Hair' scored bonus points, but the singing was atrocious! It was fun, and got the brain cells active.

The children also enjoyed a game we played at the dining room table where a correct answer to a general knowledge question allowed a step to be taken forward, and an incorrect answer meant a step back. Competition was fierce to be the first to complete a circuit of the table.

Thinking to give Riley an advantage over his older and smarter sister, Kevin asked what he thought was an easy question. "On what day of the week does Easter Friday fall, Riley?"

"Let me think. Hmmm....can you give us a few clues, Dad?"

But both our children knew, for example, that the Nile is the longest river in the world, and the Andes is a mountain range in South America, facts which they were not taught at their school. It was in this round-the-table game, too, that we taught the children suffixes and prefixes, Latin derivations, spelling, and maths tables.

Over the years, Riley established himself within the family as the creator of 'Rileyisms', a form of malapropisms whereby he misused words and sayings. His 'Rileyisms' remain part of the Brasch idiom even today, and his nieces, who were born after his death, use his expressions and attribute them to Riley.

When chosen to move a vote of thanks to some important visitors at his primary school, Riley addressed them as 'extinguished guests'! And when I dithered about how to care for my newly acquired orchids, he asked, "Didn't they give you any 'destructions' on how to care for 'awkwards'?" I always have to rely on the instructions because I do find orchids awkward to care for. Throughout the years, Riley gave consistent advice about all step-by-step operations, "If you don't know what to do, check out the destructions." Another one of Riley's little idiosyncrasies was to 'settle in'. "I'll just settle in first," he'd declare. No matter where Riley went, or for how little time he stayed, his first priority was always to 'settle in'.

"Have you settled in, Ril?" I always enquired.

"Yep, Mum, I've settled in. You've got to settle in, you know." Settling in was sacrosanct. Even when we went to the movies, we had to arrive in time to 'settle in' to our seats. Now, as a family, we can't go anywhere unless we settle in first.

We fretted endlessly about how Riley was going to make his way in life. We knew that he was 'different' and that he had trouble coping with routine tasks, but at this stage of his life, we didn't think of his problems in terms of mental illness. In the early years, we thought that being good role models for him to follow, giving him sound advice, and explaining processes would set him up well for life and help to overcome his difficulties. As well, Kevin and I had an unshakeable belief that so long as we loved him, nurtured him, and gave him opportunities and experiences that he could cope with, he would find his niche in life. Never for one second did we imagine that someone who was so loved would endure a life of such torment.

By the end of his time in Grade Three, we had come to the realisation that academia was not for Riley. There had never been any encouraging comments about his academic progress on his report cards: *Riley has a poor concentration span and does not have ready recall.* But with reference to his behaviour: *Riley tries so hard. He is always eager to please.* In an attempt to make school life as easy as possible for Riley, in his last two years of primary school, Kevin took Riley to the school where he was the Deputy Principal, and placed him in classes with teachers who had compassion for his limitations. These teachers always treated Riley with respect and understanding. Even so, Riley continued to be a misfit in the school environment.

It was at this school, though, that Riley did finally achieve one of his goals. "I'm in the team, Mum," he announced with pride. There are plenty of children who do not do well in the classroom but achieve success and the respect of their fellow students by doing well at sport. But Riley struggled both in the classroom and on the sporting field. His eye-to-hand coordination was non-existent, and when it came to choosing sides for lunchtime games or teams for school sport, Riley was at best last chosen, or more commonly, not chosen at all. Riley desperately wanted to be a member of 'the team', but his sense of worthlessness was reinforced by his regular exclusions. At all of the schools Riley attended, he was always the loner on the outside looking in at those united by team spirit.

But through the thoughtfulness of his Grade Seven teacher, only once did Riley manage to be selected as 'reserve' in the team to play football for the school, taking up a position on the wing for a brief period. At one stage during his time on the field, a good pass came his way with open ground ahead of him to score a try, but Riley didn't even raise his hands to catch the ball. He didn't seem to understand that this was what he was meant to do. Understandably, his teammates were disappointed and gave him a verbal berating.

And we thought that tennis lessons might be okay for him so we enrolled him in the school's coaching program. One day Kevin was watching, unseen, from around the corner. Riley took a good swipe at the ball, which he lobbed over the high surrounding fence and it disappeared down the oval. "Good shot, Riley," his tennis coach called encouragingly.

As well as his swimming club successes, which continued throughout his primary school years, Riley was awarded a trophy for 'The Most Improved Player' in his school's volleyball team. He always turned up for training but was never chosen to play for the school. And when he was in his early teens, he showed his physical endurance by comfortably running cross-country races for which he trained by going on long distance runs with his father. One time, he arrived home from a long run and casually said to me, "My backside is a bit sore. It's been sore for a few days."

"Can I have a look?" I asked. He had a huge boil on his bottom, but this hadn't stopped him from running twenty kilometres.

He also jogged with his father around our neighbourhood for personal fitness and in the early stages of my fitness campaign when Riley was twelve or thirteen, I started jogging at night, after work, on my own. Riley would not hear of this and insisted on accompanying me 'for safety sake', he said.

"No, I'm not protecting you, Mum. No one would want to front an old bird like you. It's the public that needs protecting. Who knows what panic might spread through the streets when people see you coming. You're scary stuff."

Nonetheless, in spite of his wry humour, he really did encourage me by setting little goals for me to run to the next streetscape feature before I collapsed to a walking pace. And he had a very simple theory that worked: "Don't look ahead, Mum. If it looks like a long way in front of you, you'll only be discouraged and give up. Look down at your feet. Just watch each step you take. One step at a time, and the distance will take care of itself." How prophetic. Our lives were destined to become one step at a time, one day at a time.

And when he spied a hill ahead, he urged, "ABH, Mum! Go for it!" Another Bloody Hill.

In those days, he was fit enough to run up and down Mt Warning twice with his father and he walked it once with me. He also went on a school excursion that involved riding bicycles throughout the South-East corner of Queensland and into Northern New South Wales. Another climb of Mt Warning was included in this trip. And during our annual holidays, Riley and his father often cycled from Tugun on the coast into the Gold Coast Hinterland.

His commitment to physical activity, however, didn't stop him from taking up smoking at an early age. Riley had been asthmatic since he was a small child, but he started smoking when he was about thirteen. I contacted the respiratory specialist who treated his asthma and asked him to have a word to Riley about the perils of smoking. Full of self-righteousness, I presented Riley for the appointment.

"So, you're smoking now Riley?" the doctor asked.

"Yes," Riley responded without a qualm.

"Why?" the doctor asked.

"I just like it," Riley replied.

"Well, I guess there are worse things that you can do," replied the doctor, and that was it. So much for words of wisdom.

Despite this setback, we tried in the following years to convince him to stop smoking. When he was a young adult, Kevin took him to other doctors who produced x-rays that revealed damage to his lungs but Riley continued to smoke. I also took him to a doctor for a bad cough, and Riley came out of the consultation with a script for nicotine chewing gum, which I purchased at great cost, but he continued to smoke and never chewed.

"Smoking's bad for your health, Ril," we told him constantly.

"Yeah?" he smirked at us. "So it kills me. Do you think that worries me?" The irony of the ills of smoking compared with the self-mutilations and suicide attempts that eventually plagued his adult life was not lost on him. In due course we conceded defeat in the face of his other, more damaging behaviour. To Riley's credit, however, we never had to ask him not to smoke in the house or in our presence. He did that automatically, as a natural act of courtesy.

Chapter 3

We had booked Riley into a large, private secondary school at birth, Kevin's alma mater, but changed this to St Jude's, a small, suburban church school, in the hope that instead of the academic and sporting competitiveness he would encounter at the original school, he would be cared for as a needy member of a Christian flock.

But at St Jude's, Riley was taunted, bullied, and physically assaulted by a particular group of students.

In his early days at this school, Riley began running away from home and deliberately cutting himself. On the first occasion that he ran away from home, he took an old scruffy blanket and spent a few hours at a nearby quarry. We were frantic and about to notify the police when he came home at dusk because, he said, the mosquitoes were biting him.

On another occasion when he ran away, the note that he left has his dried blood on it.

> *Dear Mum & Dad*
>
> *I am sorry it had to come to this but things got out of hand so I need some time to think. I will take care.*
>
> *Love always*
>
> *Ril XXXXXXXXX*

Several times during Riley's years at St Jude's, Kevin and I woke in the middle of the night to find him in the laundry, washing items of his school uniform which he had concealed from us. He had been rolled in cow dung by his tormentors.

On another occasion, his school blazer was doused in oil. I complained to his form teacher and the boys responsible were made to pay for dry cleaning. But of course, the boys only became more subversive in their taunts and torment. Consequently, not only did Riley's misery continue, but it increased because of our complaints.

I regularly arrived at the school to collect Riley, only to find him up the huge tree that shaded the parking area. He was retrieving his school bag or items of clothing thrown up the tree by the bullies.

They stood menacingly at the base of the tree, making him too terrified to come down, but they skulked off when I arrived. He also suffered severe bruising from being pushed off a school veranda into the bushes a few metres below.

Riley was so traumatised by this treatment that, as well as running away and harming himself, he began hyperventilating and once spent two days in hospital. On this occasion, he lost consciousness in the car on the way to school and Kevin thought Riley was dying. His hyperventilation became so frequent, that Kevin and I quickly learned to manage the episodes with brown paper bags and calm reassurances.

Our initial impulse was to remove Riley from St Jude's and place him in another school. We consulted Dr Stephens, a psychiatrist who specialised in the care of adolescents, and he advised against this. "You might be taking him out of the frying pan and putting him in the fire," he cautioned. How could we guarantee that Riley would not encounter the same treatment at another school let alone cope with the difficulty that abruptly changing schools would cause a timid boy like Riley?

Riley was also exhibiting angry behaviour towards us. Attempting to dispel my anguish about this, Dr Stephens explained, "You know that song 'You Always Hurt the One You Love?' Why do you think they wrote that? Riley vents his anger and hurts you because he knows your love for him is secure. He knows you won't stop loving him just because he does things that distresses you." There was an irony in the doctor's reference to this song because Riley was familiar with it. When it played on my Mills Bros tape, he always said, "That Hugh's a bad bugger, Mum."

"Why is that, Ril?" I would ask.

"Well, it says 'Hugh always hurt the one you love'. What do you reckon Hugh did to have a song written about whatever it is that he does?"

When we gave Dr Stephens background information about Riley's verbal skills but lack of ability to perform tasks, he informed us that the high achievements of Kevin, Coby, and myself were detrimental to Riley's estimation of his own worth and position in our family. Although Riley was unreservedly proud that his father, mother, and sister excelled at whatever they undertook, he was convinced that he let the family down because of his inability to do likewise.

"If Riley had been born into a family of dirt-poor, uneducated onion farmers, where nothing more challenging than driving a tractor up and down a furrow confronted him each day, he would probably be okay," advised the doctor.

What were we to do? Radically alter our lives? Cease to succeed? It was an appalling dilemma, and there were many times when I was on the verge of resigning from my job and giving up study to devote my time entirely to Riley. But I knew that would be foolish and damaging to both of us. I would be martyring myself, and Riley's quest for independence would be compromised. He didn't want to be an appendage of his parents, a 'veggie' to use one of Riley's self-descriptors, propped up by his mummy and daddy. He wanted to make his own way in life, to decide his own decides.

Dr Stephens continued, "He's an angry young man who needs a few guidelines about anger management. It's not unusual in teenagers. Growing up is fraught with difficulty and the odds are somewhat stacked against Riley." But there was never an actual diagnosis, never a name put to what it was that troubled Riley.

Throughout the period of Riley's illness, and especially in the later years of his mental incapacity, the medical profession failed him with either glib diagnoses or misjudging the seriousness of his mental health. It wasn't until after Riley died that a psychiatrist said to me, "Your son was seriously ill."

For two years, until Riley was almost fourteen, we visited Dr Stephens' smart consulting rooms high above the city skyline. I took great comfort from his advice and empathy, but Riley continued to behave in a dysfunctional manner. By now, he was running away from home regularly and frequently cutting his arms and legs. We couldn't reason with him and his rages were seething, hissing confrontations.

While Riley was at St Jude's, he had plastic surgery to pin his ears back in the hope that his self-image would improve, and also to remedy a physical feature that was the brunt of teasing. It was during this time, too, that Riley needed orthodontic treatment, but this resulted in other episodes of bizarre behaviour.

"Call me Tony," the orthodontist invited Riley at the first consultation. "With the treatment you require, we are going to have a very long association. So let's skip the formalities and go straight to first names from the start. You'll be a young man by the time I finish with your mouth and we'll be old mates." And the treatment was going to cost thousands of dollars. Bands were fitted, appliances were made, and of course dental hygiene was of the utmost importance.

"Brushed your teeth, Riley?" I asked as he was going to bed. Eventually, I became aware of time passing, and odd noises coming from the bathroom. When I went to see what was happening, I found Riley brushing frenetically. His gums were pulped, blood was everywhere, and all the bands were sprung.

"What are you doing? Stop it! Stop!" I shouted, grabbing his hand to wrest the toothbrush from him.

"You want me to brush my teeth? Well, I've brushed my teeth. Satisfied?" He snarled at me.

It was difficult to explain to Tony how and why Riley's mouth and bands were reduced to this state, but after this sort of thing happened a few more times, we gave up on orthodontics.

Early in Riley's time at St Jude's when we became aware of the bullying he was enduring, we took our complaints to the Headmaster, Mr Donovan.

"No, no, no, I can't accept what you are claiming," he protested. "The boys at this school are fine lads from good families and I don't believe any of them would be unkind to another student. We're a small school with a good spirit, you know. You must be mistaken." We assured him that we were not mistaken. "Well, if what you say is true, and I seriously doubt that it is," he went on, "well, it's all part of growing up, isn't it?" No, we could not agree with him. He continued, "If anything is going on, I think we should leave it to the boys to sort out among themselves. We're not in the business of molly-coddling the boys."

"But Mr Donovan, there is a group of bullies and Riley is on his own," we responded. "How do you suggest he goes about sorting that out? That's the crux of his problem. He can't sort it out."

"Don't you think it might be timely for your lad to learn some coping skills? He needs to toughen up. This could be a character building exercise for him, don't you think? Anyhow, if it pleases you, I'll make some discreet inquiries."

Mostly, he spoke to us over his shoulder as he moved around his office doing little tidying chores. He put books on shelves, taking great care to make sure they were in the appropriate place. Then he sorted through sheets of paper, briefly scanning them, and placing them in trays or folders.

We persisted even though he was glancing at his watch. We told him about the disappearance of six of Kevin's collectable football jerseys. We found out that Riley had boasted to the boys about his father's jersey collection in the hope that he might win some acceptance, but the boys used threats to intimidate him to take the jerseys and distribute them to the group. Riley thought the jerseys would buy protection, which would free him from the violence he endured daily.

But Mr Donovan was not interested in Kevin's jerseys. "That's a private matter for you to deal with – it's got nothing to do with this school," he said, flapping his hand at us in a gesture of dismissal. Later, we contacted the boys' families but only one jersey was returned. The other parents were not concerned about the circumstances of the jerseys coming into their sons' possession and kept them.

Finally, Mr Donovan announced that he had other matters to attend to and our meeting was terminated without any resolution. Mr Donovan's 'discreet' inquiries resulted in no action being taken against Riley's tormentors and his misery continued.

Kevin and I cried many times at the cruelty we knew Riley was enduring.

Two weeks before Riley died, he told me the names of the boys at St Jude's who were his most persistent tormentors, but I didn't recognise them.

"The worst years of my life were the ones I spent at Jude's. Did you know that, Mum?" He named five or six boys. "They did things to me that I have nightmares about. It's all inside my head. It stuffs me up."

"Like what, son?"

"No, you don't need to know. What's done is done and you can't change it." He faced me and grabbed hold of my shoulders, looking me straight in the eyes. This was a familiar gesture of reassurance from Riley. He continued, "But it was worse than everything else in my life. I wish I could forget."

"I know some things, Riley. Your dad and I went to see Mr Donovan. Remember? What else happened, Riley? Tell me, please?"

"I can't, Mum. I just want to forget. I shouldn't have said anything. It's bad enough that I still have nightmares about that place. Let's just drop it."

For me, there is more torment in imagining than in knowing.

It was obvious to me that both the school and these particular boys played a significant role in Riley's mental health, and his eventual death. So much for being held within the caring folds of a Christian community.

Many years later, when Riley was a private psychiatric patient, he wrote in his diary about his time at St Jude's:

> *using writing as a release mechanism is good this is why im starting my diary especiacely tonight I have had about 12 years of living through hell and I cant understand why my parents have also lived the same agony. even as I write this my blood is boiling and it is 11.05 at night the stress running through me is over wellming I feel i'm looking at my self through my own eyes and racing at me are my ugly years. My ugly years started when I was 12 as a school kid getting bashed every day this continued every day for 3 years. My teenageed years were hell having bad acne didn't help my cause I left my first 3 years of hell at 16 a real mess.*

At the end of his Year Ten, we removed Riley from St Jude's and enrolled him in a training course offered by a small Catholic school. The course was a one-year, non-academic program for boys who had difficulties with mainstream academia. Fewer than twenty boys were enrolled in the course, which taught practical life-skills and gave the boys real-life experience with aspects of blue-collar employment. The curriculum should have offered excellent opportunities for personal growth and development, but in reality it didn't improve Riley's situation much from his experiences at St Jude's.

"Stand up, Simpson. Oh, you are standing," was one of Brother Paul's favourite jokes, said repeatedly in front of student and parent groups. Simpson always cringed. But Brother Paul persisted with his gibes. Brother Paul was in charge of the program and he appeared to take great pleasure in using sarcasm to constantly belittle the boys. He seemed to have an agenda of breaking the boys down with criticism rather than developing their self-esteem and confidence with praise.

In the first month of Riley's year in this course, Coby was seriously ill, and we were all concerned for her. Riley always became extremely distressed if any misfortune befell his beloved family. Kevin wrote a letter to Brother Paul explaining the situation and asked that Riley be given some leeway on assignments. But there was no response or any sympathetic inquiry, and Brother Paul's expectations of Riley's daily performance were demanding even though he was distraught.

Part of the course curriculum required the boys to do volunteer work for a needy or charitable organisation for half a day each week and to get paid, part-time employment for one day of the school week. In a strange twist of fate, Riley's volunteer work was in the geriatric annex of the hospital where he was soon to become a psychiatric patient. He loved working with the old folk, especially when they had music therapy, and the skills he gained handling wheelchairs allowed him to take command of his adored grandmother's wheelchair. "You don't go up and down gutters like that, Mum. You'll tip her out. Here, let me show you," he said as he elbowed me away from the wheelchair. And my mother would say whenever Riley was with us, "Riley will wheel me, thank you." She trusted him.

He obtained part-time work with a ships' chandlery, repairing shipping containers. He off-sided for the welders, and safety glasses were essential protective equipment for the eyes. But he regularly got metal shavings in his eyes. We had to take him to an eye specialist several times to have metal fragments removed. Obviously, he was not wearing eye protection, but his reason for not doing so was that his face was so small, none of the available safety glasses fitted him. To overcome this, we took him to an optometrist to have his own safety glasses custom made, but within hours of collecting them, he wilfully destroyed them as an act of self-punishment. He never saw himself as being worthy of such precautions.

At the end of his year in the training course, we were no closer to finding Riley's elusive niche in life. And as he was now on the brink of adulthood and about to add the burden of finding a job to his difficulties, Kevin and I had mixed emotions of hope and fear.

In these early years of his self-harm, we hid any instruments or implements that we thought Riley could use to hurt himself. We regularly slept with knives and blades, even screwdrivers, hidden under our pillows. I hid all of my kitchen knives throughout the house and once sent my sister to the broom cupboard to retrieve the bread knife. Of course she thought this was a bit odd, but that was how I had to manage sharp instruments in the home.

To stop him from running away, we slept with the keys to the house under our pillows, too, so that Riley couldn't abscond at night. However, with the passage of time, the sheer futility of our efforts eventually became patently obvious as we gradually realised that we were no match for the mental torment that drove him to such behaviour. As dedicated as we were to removing all weapons that Riley might use to harm himself, he was just as dedicated to circumventing our efforts. Eventually, we stopped hiding things, and braced ourselves for the inevitable outcomes.

As he got older, his sudden departures from home became more regular. Sometimes he left a note, but mostly, he just disappeared.

Kevin and I looked for him for days, taking time off from work. We searched the nearby bush calling his name. We prowled city streets and lanes. We searched under bridges, and every nook and cranny of Brisbane's Expo site. We made phone calls to people and places that we knew he associated with, and of course, we reported his disappearances to the police, but they took little interest in his disappearances, and never once found him when he was missing.

Chapter 4

When Riley finished school, Kevin and I hoped that he could leave these traumatic years behind him, find a job, and get on with his life in a positive way. But his erratic behaviour continued and our concern for him deepened. For the first few years of his mental turmoil, we tried to find answers and treatment through private practitioners. Although he cut himself often, his wounds were usually superficial but one day, he cut himself so badly, we had to rush him to a local doctor to have the wound stitched. This doctor referred us to a nearby public mental health unit.

At last, I thought. A sense of relief washed over me. Now we'll get help. They'll see that Riley is ill and treat him. Someone will help us. Surely that's what a psychiatric hospital is for. This was our first encounter with the public mental health system. Riley was sixteen.

After being assessed at the unit, Riley was hospitalised for a few days. But there was no particular outcome to his stay, and I was disappointed and confused. My expectations of the hospital had not eventuated. I soon realised that I was naive in my anticipation of how the public mental health system would treat Riley. Although Riley did receive intermittent treatment over the next six or seven years at this unit, there never seemed to be a consistent, overall plan or continuity of treatment for him. Treatment always appeared to be ad hoc, depending on which roster of medical staff was on duty at the time.

Throughout the years, I was interviewed several times by primary care nurses who were new to Riley's case, and it was apparent to me that they were not aware of his history. With each new primary care nurse, we seemed to start at the beginning again. The same old questions were asked, and I gave the same old answers.

"I've been through all this before," I would tell them. "Isn't all of this in his notes, his medical history?" It seemed to me that his treatment plan was static, rather than progressive. I was frustrated and I despaired.

Because of Riley's escalating self-harm, he was regularly admitted to hospitals all over Brisbane. He roamed to all points of the compass around Brisbane, and when the police or the ambulance became involved in his injuries, they took him to the nearest public psychiatric unit. But as soon as his wounds were treated and the legal requirement of seventy-two hours detention had elapsed, he would be released without on-going treatment for the underlying cause of his injuries — his mental state. Sometimes, he was not even detained for the seventy-two hours, like the time he was treated in the Accident and Emergency Department of one large public hospital after swallowing a safety razor. They removed the razor surgically and sent him home. This hospital has a large psychiatric unit attached, but Riley was not admitted to it, nor was his mental state investigated.

Eventually, when this sort of thing was happening regularly, we sought an appointment with the medical director of one of these mental health units. At first, we were told that the medical director, a senior psychiatrist, was too busy to meet with us. But we persisted because we were unyielding in our belief that Riley needed long-term psychiatric treatment and not just detention, or worse still, emergency repairs to his physical damage, and then discharge without any psychiatric assessment. Eventually, we were granted an appointment, but instead of meeting with just the doctor assigned to Riley's case, we were confronted by twelve medical administrators. This consisted of senior and junior psychiatrists, case managers, and social workers. We were meant to be intimidated, and we were. This meeting wasn't about Riley's welfare. It was a power play meant to leave Kevin and me in no doubt that we had no right to question the public mental health system. One senior staff member dominated the meeting and conveyed a clear message to us: 'How dare you question what we are doing.'

After this meeting, a young doctor followed us into the corridor. Dr Mah introduced himself and ushered us around the corner, away from the scrutiny of his superiors.

"Mr and Mrs Brasch, can I have a moment? Please let me apologise for the way you were treated in there. I'm so upset. It was just terrible. I'm only a junior staff member, just observing processes.

You are right about Riley needing more extensive treatment than we are providing. But you are not going to get that here, in the public system, so please, do look elsewhere for treatment. The administration's hopeless and heartless. I wish you and Riley well. Please phone me if you think I can be of any help." He wrote his details on a piece of paper before darting off furtively, lest he be seen talking with us.

The following day, one of the social workers who had been present at the meeting also phoned to apologise for our treatment, as well as Riley's, and she too encouraged us to seek further treatment outside the public health system.

Ultimately, there was no effective treatment within the public mental health system for Riley. They merely patched him up and complied with their legal obligation. In current circumstances, there is little hope for proper treatment of many mental patients in the public system.

Riley's situation was not unique. According to *Dare to care: SANE Mental Health Report 2004:* 'Mental health services are in crisis to varying degrees all around Australia, barely able to cope with people experiencing acute episodes of illness, let alone provide ongoing treatment and support.' The report continues: 'The symptoms [of mental illness] and disability experienced cause profound distress for those affected and their families. Untreated, or ineffectively treated, it is a major contributor to the high suicide rate in our country.'

The Royal Australian and New Zealand College of Psychiatrists claims that mentally ill people who are discharged from hospital too early account for almost half of Queensland's 25,000 homeless people because there is nowhere else for them to go, except the streets. Safe hostel accommodation, or preferably, supported accommodation is almost non-existent. This exposes them to street violence, crime, and they are more likely to contract illnesses, other than their existing mental illness, because of rough living conditions and the inability to access services.

Despite contemporary policies of deinstitutionalisation and community integration, founded on humane and innovative philosophies, branch member of the RANZCP, Dr Josey Sundin claims that: "Past policies of deinstitutionalisation of the mentally ill had been economically misused by governments. They took money out of institutions and have never put it back into the community." This has led to a reduction of inpatient treatment, services provided by community health centres, and an absence of vital support once patients are thrust into the outside world. Riley was told on discharge on one occasion: "It's time you took responsibility for yourself." This was tantamount to expecting a man with two broken legs to run a marathon. The result of these reductions in service is that many psychiatric patients are in a state of crisis, unable to cope, and for some of them, the outcomes are tragic.

Compounding the inadequacy of the mental health system, support resources, and accommodation options, is the attitude of many people within our society. Ostracism, stigma, bigotry, and fear of the mentally ill thrives within our so-called egalitarian communities, effectively thwarting any hope for the Rileys of this world to blend in with 'normal' people.

In his Symposium 2003 address titled, 'Out of the Darkness', President of the Schizophrenia Fellowship of New South Wales, Judge Frank Walker said it is an unfortunate reality that, with regard to mental illness, 'when you scratch the veneer of modern society many…primitive beliefs still lurk beneath the surface'. Riley struggled to move beyond this prejudice and achieve the normal aspects of life that are taken for granted by the majority of the population. He wanted the freedom to decide his own decides, the dignity and material benefits that employment brings, respect for his achievements, good mates, a girlfriend – perhaps a family, and medical treatment that met his needs. His hopes and aspirations were not unreasonable but they *were* unattainable.

A psychiatric nurse from one of the public hospitals where Riley was being detained referred us to yet another psychologist whose speciality was the inter-relatedness of family relationships and adolescence. He gave his diagnosis in Riley's presence: "There's no pathology to indicate a mental illness. He's just being a little bastard, behaving as he does. He needs to smarten up, get his act together, and you need to take a strong hand with his discipline. Don't put up with what he's dishing out. Take a stand. You need to think of the family unit, not just this badly behaved individual."

My son a bastard? I was stunned, unable to comprehend that a professional practitioner from whom we were seeking guidance would not only assess my son in this manner, but do it in Riley's presence.

Many years later, Riley remembered that he had been labelled a bastard and wrote this letter to us:

> *Dear Mum and Dad,*
>
> *Firstly I would like to thank you for the visit wich included your self and dad, to wynum. I really had a good time. This visit was our last one. The reason I havenot phoned you is because thic is the way it will be from now on. No moore visits ore phone calls from now on, and there is no negotiation. I am no longer a part of the Brasch family, my new family consists of Hilery as my mother, and Jesus as my father. finally i would like to thank you for putting up with such a BARSTARD of a son but life must go on. I hold both of you in high regard and that is all I can say*
>
> *Yours Fathfully*
>
> *Riley Brasch.*

Hilary was the landlady of one of the better hostels in Brisbane where Riley lived intermittently. He was fond of this kind and gentle woman. His reference to Jesus would have been made to rankle his father and me because he knew we were non-believers. Despite our lack of faith, though, both of our children had attended Sunday School as youngsters and they were educated at church secondary schools. And we had a commitment through the children's bedtime routine to give them the opportunity to accept God into their lives if they chose to do so. When Riley was a little fellow his bedtime routine always included a simple prayer asking God to keep him safe and well, to help him to be honest and thoughtful, to bless those whom he loved, and to help others who might be in need of His benevolence. Then we finished off with this child's verse:

The tiny rabbits play no more,
The little birds are weary.
The buttercups are folded up,
Good night, good night, my deary.

The children in the country,
And the children in the city,
Are off to bed with nodding heads,
Good night, good night, my pretty.

After this, we would have a chat about whatever was relevant at the time. During these chats, he often told me, "Mummy, I would like to be a minister when I grow up."

"Why, Ril?" I would ask.

"I want to be kind to people and help them. That's what ministers do, you know," he replied earnestly.

"You can be what ever you set your heart on, my love," I promised him. "If you really want something, you *can* make it happen. Your Daddy and I will do everything we can to help you achieve your dreams."

When did ambition die and our hope fade?

Much later, when Riley was in his late teens, we had a lengthy discussion about religion. He was keen to know why I disbelieved. I explained my theories on religion to him. He was pensive and asked probing questions.

"But you don't have to have the same opinions as I do, Riley," I assured him. "You need to think about your own values and ideas on religion and follow whatever means something to you or gives you comfort. My opinions do not have to be your opinions. Do what you always do, son, and decide your own decides."

We had encouraged the children to think about the issues of faith and make their own decisions. Earlier, in one of his forays into independence, Riley had dabbled for a short period with Catholicism but eventually decided that this belief system was not for him. It was while Riley was experimenting with the values of the Catholic Church that one lot of flatmates he was sharing accommodation with took him shopping for suits that he could not afford so that he could attend church on Sunday evenings. But Riley was the only one at church in a suit on the hot summer evenings. The suits were too big for him as well. He also had purchased an assortment of ill-fitting shirts and ties that his grandfather would have worn. What use are suits to a person who spends most of his days in psychiatric hospitals? But at least he pleased his new friends, who probably had a good laugh at him.

A few weeks after our chat he said to me, "I've given a lot of thought to what we talked about, you know, about religion, and I'm with you, Mum. I can't believe in all that religious stuff. It's mumbo jumbo if you ask me. If there really is a loving God, why is He letting all this rubbish happen in our lives? And if there is a life after death and a heaven, Poppy (his late grandfather) would look down on us and make things right, wouldn't he? Poppy would look after us if he could, but that hasn't happened. I don't believe that there is anything except what happens here on earth."

Riley's reasoning was simple, less reproachful than mine. I remember once driving away from the hospital, in tears, overwhelmed by sorrow. On this visit to Riley, he dispassionately demonstrated to me how easily he could hang himself from the curtain rail around his bed. "But they keep coming in to check on me. I'm on five-minute observations. They don't give me enough time to do it. I wish they'd bloody-well drop off and give me a chance," he complained.

As I drove home, the vision of his demonstration played over and over in my head. 'Why did my son desire death instead of loving life?' I interrogated myself. I started thumping the steering wheel. Tears blurred my vision. The thought went through my mind that if there was a God, instead of saying 'Suffer the little children to come unto Me,' when He looked at Riley He simply said, 'Suffer.' And suffer Riley did. No kind and loving God ever watched over Riley.

As we continued to search for answers about Riley's mental state, another psychologist counselled me.

"Mrs Brasch, I don't know what to advise you. This is a terrible situation for you and your son. It's beyond me to know a way forward. I'm happy to work with Riley on issues of anger management and the difficulties of being a teenager, but I think he needs much more than that. You both need assistance. I wish I could be more helpful."

I was grateful for this psychologist's frankness, but I still wanted to know what was wrong with my son.

We spent years trawling through psychiatric and psychology consulting rooms in Brisbane seeking help for Riley. We also pursued community organisations that we heard provided training and support programs for troubled teenagers, but when Kevin and I met with the organisers, it became apparent that Riley's difficulties fell outside their area of expertise.

We felt alone and isolated in dealing with what troubled Riley. It seemed to us that no one understood our plight and no one could help us. No doubt, Riley felt this more intensely than we did.

Chapter 5

"I've got a job, Mum. I got it all by myself. I'll be driving a forklift in a supermarket warehouse. I start next Monday." Riley's excitement was infectious.

In an attempt to boost Riley's employment prospects, Kevin had worked hard with him to attain a forklift licence through the Technical and Further Education program.

"That's great, son. Well done."

For the first week, Riley's joy at being employed bubbled over. In the mornings, he was out of bed early, keen to get to work. In the evenings, he chatted animatedly about his duties, the other blokes, and the trivia of the workplace.

Early in the second week, I detected a drop in his mood.

"How was work today?" I asked.

"Good. They're moving me around. Trying me out in different sections. Seeing where I fit in best." I had heard variations of this before.

By the middle of the second week, he was more despondent.

"There's talk in the lunch room that some blokes are going to be laid off. Not enough business to keep all of us on the job. Last on, first off. That's the routine. And I'm last on." I'd heard this before, too.

I knew that it was not possible, but I wished that I could go to his workplace, seek out his superior, and beg him to keep Riley on the job. Find something for him to do. There must be something he can do. Anything. Please. I knew how important employment was for Riley's self-esteem. There is dignity in being employed, and Riley needed a solid dose of dignity.

By Friday, Riley was unemployed.

"I was last on, Mum. So if they had to let people go, I was first to get my marching orders. They said they'd contact me when they were putting people on again." But he never heard from them. Yet again, his excitement at getting the job was replaced by his dejection at being dismissed.

Every time Riley was employed, according to him, the firm had to let people go within the first two weeks, and 'last on, first off' was a familiar mantra for Riley.

The one time when Riley didn't invoke the 'last on, first off' excuse was when he got a job with a company that maintained the nature strips along major roads. About three weeks into the job, Riley was sacked for filling the tank of a diesel truck with petrol. "It wasn't even my job to refuel the trucks," he told me. "Marty was late so I thought I'd do it for him. You know, show a bit of initiative. Make a good impression. I didn't know it was a diesel truck, Mum. I just wanted to be helpful."

For a year or so, Riley worked intermittently as a casual labourer in a canning factory. He wasn't fussed on the job, but he must have been well thought of because after he had failed to report for work for a few weeks, his supervisor phoned our home asking after him and encouraging us to persuade Riley to return to the job. He did, but his heart was never in it and he had some difficulties during this time, least of all because he got upset when there were police raids to flush out illegal immigrants.

He rode his bicycle to and from the factory, and one day on the way home, he fell off and broke his shoulder. On another occasion, he cut the palm of his hand badly and required over ten stitches. He wasn't living at home at the time, and two weeks after the accident, we called at his accommodation to take him on an outing. He hadn't been back to the doctor to have the stitches removed and his hand was puffed up like a balloon with infection. He was in extreme pain, but seemed to think that this was how things should be. He refused our pleading to return to the doctor. Finally, we had to physically force him to the surgery of a friend who had a difficult task locating the stitches, which were deeply embedded in proud flesh.

It was at the factory that he met David.

Riley had come back to live at home, at this time. His living arrangements were like Melbourne's weather — unpredictable on a daily basis. During this stay, I became aware of regular phone calls in the evenings, and Riley's abrupt, monosyllabic responses. After the calls, he paced around the house, agitated, tense, uncommunicative.

"Who was that, Ril?"

"No one you know."

"What did they want?"

"Nothing."

"So they just phoned to say nothing?"

"Get off my case, Mum."

"Just trying to help, son."

"Give it a rest, okay?"

"Fine. Whatever, Ril."

It was the same routine for the next few nights. Kevin was away, so I knew I had to sort out whatever was worrying Riley. On the fourth night, I beat Riley to the phone.

"Who am I speaking to?" I enquired.

"Can I speak to Riley?"

"No, you can't. You'll speak to me. You've been phoning here every night this week. What do you want?"

"Do yourself a favour lady, and put Riley on. I don't want to speak to you."

"You do yourself a favour, mate, and tell me who you are and what you want."

I was aware of Riley pacing behind me, throwing his arms around, babbling.

"God, you've done it now, Mum! You've bloody done it now! You haven't got a clue, have you? Bloody hell!"

Back to the caller.

"He owes me $800 and I want it. Now."

"And why would Riley owe you $800?"

"It's a loan I gave him to take to the track. I want it back now."

"You can't mean the racetrack?" I laughed. "Riley's not a gambler. He wouldn't know how to bet and he wouldn't know one end of a horse from the other."

"Listen, lady. I don't give a shit if he doesn't know a horse's arse from its head, but he owes me $800. Are you his mother? Listen closely, lady. I know where you live. If you're smart, you'll get your boy cashed up to give me my money back."

"I am not prepared to continue this conversation. When I find out what your name is, I'll be reporting you to the police. You're an extortionist, and extortion is a crime, so, if *you're* smart, you won't phone here again!"

After the call, I interrogated Riley. He confirmed the circumstances of the debt. Yes, he did owe this person $800. He had borrowed it to take to the racetrack to impress a prospective friend. Of course he lost all of the money, and now he had no hope of repaying it.

The following night, the caller phoned again, but with a conciliatory tone.

"Hello, Mrs Brasch. My name is David Friend. I think we got off to a bad start last night." I almost laughed at the irony of his name. He continued, "I'm hoping we can come to some arrangement about Riley's debt. I'm out of work, I'm behind in the rent, my girlfriend is pregnant, and I really need my money back."

"Well, Mr Friend, it wasn't very bright of you to lend someone like Riley such a large amount of money, was it?"

"No. I know that now. But I did. And I want my money back. And you know that word you called me…."

"What word?"

"Something you called me. You said it was a crime and you'd phone the police about it?"

"Extortionist? You mean extortionist?"

"Yes, ex….extort…. I asked someone what it meant, and I'm not an…whatever that word is. Riley asked me for the money. I gave it to him in good faith. Tell you what. If you repay the money quickly, I'll take $600 as a done deal."

Whoever had advised Mr Friend about the meaning of the word extortionist, may also have advised him on the wisdom of making a good deal for both parties, and being polite.

The next day, I put $600 in the bank account nominated by Mr Friend, and he phoned to thank me when he had access to the money. I think I liked him. We had both tried to talk tough, but neither of us really was.

This was only one of many times when we had to rescue Riley from financial disasters, but none of Riley's creditors endeared themselves to me quite like Mr Friend.

In one of Riley's many attempts at independence, he found accommodation in Shorncliffe but within weeks he fell behind in his rent and was informed by his landlord that if the arrears were not paid by five o'clock that afternoon, he would be evicted. Kevin and I wanted to pay his outstanding rent, but Riley resisted.

"Let me fix it," he pleaded. "I have got some backbone, you know. I can do some things for myself." He was unemployed at the time, on the dole, and he knew that Social Security issued emergency funds for situations such as this.

Although he wouldn't allow us to pay his rent, he did agree that I could accompany him to the Social Security office in case he ran into bureaucratic procedures that he didn't understand, but I was instructed to 'keep my bib out of things'. I was there under sufferance.

We went there in the morning and made a successful application for emergency funds and were then informed that we had to return to the office that afternoon, when the cheques would be issued.

When we came back, about fifteen other people were waiting for cheques as well. I sat back trying to be inconspicuous, but I could hear conversations about hardship around me.

"My kids have gone to school today hungry," said a dad. "There's no food in the house. I need this cheque to buy food for tea tonight, or they'll go to bed hungry as well. I've promised them fish and chips. They love fish and chips."

"I've got no nappies for my baby, and the formula is almost gone, too," said a young mother, clutching a bunny-rugged infant to her.

"My little girl's got asthma," another young mother added. "I need to get her a puffer from the chemist."

I felt guilty because I had cash in my handbag. I wanted to run out and buy nappies and groceries, but I continued to sit quietly, to watch and listen.

Time passed and those around me were becoming restless. At three o'clock, a man went to the counter and rapped on it. "Excuse me. Excuse me, please. We were told to be here at two o'clock. It's nearly three now. When will we get our cheques?"

"You'll get them when they're ready," snapped the staff member, who turned on his heel to return to the back of the office.

I could see staff at the back, having afternoon tea. They were chatting and laughing, oblivious to our concerns.

"I could smarten this lot up, Ril," I told him.

"Don't you dare, Mum," he warned. "You sit tight and keep your mouth shut."

A half hour later, a young woman went to the counter. She caught the eye of one of the staff. "The bank closes at four o'clock. How much longer do we have to wait?"

She got the same indifferent reply, as the chatting among the staff continued.

Finally, Riley had his say. "We were told to be here at two o'clock. It's now nearly four. The banks close at four. What's going on?"

"Please sit down and be patient. Your inquiries are only causing delays."

"We've been bloody patient for two hours!" Riley exploded.

"Sir, there is no need to be rude. Please sit down. You are causing delays," admonished the woman.

At three minutes to four, a staff member strolled to the counter with a string of cheques in his hand. As he tore them off, he called names: Anderson. Biggs. Brasch. Jones. Murphy. He was casual and unhurried as desperate hands grabbed their cheques and began running to the bank, which was about two hundred metres down the mall.

I watched a mother drag a toddler along the road as she ran to get to the bank before it closed, but the toddler couldn't keep up with her, so she dragged him, screaming.

The young mother with the infant who needed nappies tried to run while clutching the baby to her.

Others ran like stampeding cattle with a scent of water in their nostrils.

The bank must have been accustomed to this spectacle each afternoon, because a young bank employee stood at the door, holding it open. He seemed unfazed by the desperate procession. "Don't run. We'll hold the door open for you all. You'll get your cheques cashed." He pulled the fallen toddler up with his free hand.

I couldn't believe this had happened.

Following his demoralising attempts at employment, Riley's sole source of income for many years was from the dole, and in the last three or four years of his life, from a Disability Support Pension. Once he got the pension, he announced, "I'm going to buy a town house, Mum. In Coorparoo. I like Coorparoo."

"Really?" I asked. "How are you going to afford that, Riley?"

"Well, with that rental allowance that I'm going to get now, I'll be able to buy a unit. It will set me up for life."

Because Riley was living away from home, he was also entitled to a rental allowance of $71.45 a fortnight. Riley sincerely believed that the extra money would make him financially secure, and able to purchase property. But when I showed him on paper that his income was insufficient to finance a mortgage, he became agitated.

"You don't want me to get ahead," he accused. "You're stuffing up all my dreams."

What Kevin and I tried to do as the mayhem of Riley's life escalated was to coax him to be organised and have a daily routine. We naively thought that an ordered life would result in an ordered mind. I put a white board in his bedroom so that he could write up both short- and long-term tasks. And I wanted Riley to take an active role in his finances. Every week I helped him to prepare a budget so that necessities were purchased, he had some cash in his pocket for enjoyment, and savings were put aside for the future. But in reality, I was the only one participating in these processes. Everything that I said or did was forgotten or ignored by Riley in the instant that I stopped speaking. It was not a wilful action on his behalf, but the way his brain malfunctioned. And with the despair that he lived with daily, he didn't see the point in planning ahead.

Responding to letters of demand and phone calls from businesses and landlords to whom Riley owed money became such a demanding part of my daily routine, I eventually took over full management of his meagre income so that it was used appropriately and bad debts were avoided. Riley had no interest whatsoever in financial responsibility, nor was he bothered about the role I took in his finances. The greatest difficulty Riley had with money was that he had no understanding its value, of the difference between one dollar, ten dollars, or one hundred dollars. It was all the same to him and might as well have been Monopoly money. If he had cash in his pocket, it didn't last long and its dispersal could never be accounted for, and there was never any tangible evidence of how he had spent his money. But I was meticulous in keeping all records relating to Riley's funds.

Apart from the challenge of trying to keep Riley's finances in good order, I spent a considerable amount of time every day making his Medicare claims. His claims on Medicare were confusing because of his complicated health history and his ever-changing addresses. In any short period of his adult life, he could be living at home, dossing down in low-rent accommodation, living in a hostel, or he could just be 'missing', living rough on the road. Where he was at the start of each day had no correlation with where his day ended.

But it wasn't only his living arrangements that were complex. So too was his medical history. He could start the day in a private hospital but end it in a public facility. Or every possible combination of all the options. His impulsive behaviour could change his circumstances in an instant. His life was in constant disarray.Because of this, I was never sure which box I should tick for the questions on the Medicare form about inpatient and outpatient treatment and I never knew what to write in the 'Change of Address' section. And it took regular phone sessions with Marion, from the Queensland Ambulance Service, to track Riley's use of the service: "Have I claimed for this one? Where was he picked up from for that ride? Which hospital did he go to on that day?"

"Hold on," Marion would say. "Let's start from the beginning again. I'll list them, and you cross them off."

Eventually, Kevin and I were summonsed on Riley's behalf to meet with a Medicare administrator in the city office to discuss his situation. After explaining Riley's complex medical and accommodation history, I was directed to send his claims to one particular assessor who, it was hoped, now had an understanding of Riley's copious and convoluted claims. The administrator even printed off a few sheets of address labels to assist me.

More often than not, I didn't have an account to start with, but if I knew that Riley had received some recent medical treatment, I rang around to find out where he had been, if any money was owed, and whether there was a follow-up appointment or whatever. It was a constant challenge, but I made many friends with faceless voices on the phone. We were united in a quest to sort out Riley's financial affairs: they wanted their accounts paid, and I wanted to keep him solvent.

One of the things that my financial management achieved for Riley was to allow him to purchase his own car.

Apart from his desire to have his driver's licence and own a car, Kevin and I were also keen for Riley to achieve these milestones to bolster his self-esteem and boost his employment opportunities. When he was seventeen, he passed the test for his driver's licence at his first attempt. As well as the professional driving lessons that we gave him for his seventeenth birthday, Kevin augmented the lessons with plenty of driving practice and tutoring him on the road rules. They were both overjoyed at their success and we thought that it was an amazing achievement for Riley.

Initially, Riley couldn't afford a car so, until enough of his small income was saved, we bought him a zippy little motor scooter to get him to and from occasional casual work. Then when he was twenty-one, the car became a reality.

"You've got enough money saved, Ril, to buy your own car," I told him.

"But we've been to all the Used Car Yards, Mum, and anything decent costs more than I've got in the bank. I want a good car. I don't want a lemon." Riley and I had spent many weekends window-shopping at car yards.

"Well, your father has decided to upgrade the Corona. It's in excellent condition and you know its history. You can have it for what you've got saved. It's a good deal if you think the Corona is the car for you. What do you say?"

"Yeah! Great! Sounds good to me! How soon can we do the deal?" he enthused.

A few weeks later, we handed him the keys to the Corona. We made a ceremony of it with handshakes and photos. "Wow!" he said. "My own car! I never thought I would ever own a car!"

However, any notions that Kevin and I had about Riley appreciating and respecting the car were futile. He allowed so-called friends to drive his car, and it became their street-racer. On one occasion, the car was bogged in a council park for several days and Riley was issued with a notice to remove it. It was so badly bogged, Kevin couldn't shift it. When he tried to get our car close enough to tow Riley's out, our car became bogged, too. Finally, it developed into a major undertaking to remove Ril's car, involving a professional tow truck.

There was also the girlfriend of one of the street-racers who persuaded Riley to let her use his car to practice her driving skills. She bunny-hopped up and down the street, grated the gears, and scraped the tyres on the gutter. Although Riley knew that what was happening to his car was wrong, he was afraid of losing friendships if he didn't volunteer his car for these escapades.

He also used the car as a place of isolation where he could indulge in his ever-increasing habit of self-mutilation. He carved *Death* and *Devil* on his forearm and legs with a blade, and matched this with the same carvings on the leather of the steering wheel and front instrument panel.

Within six months, we paid $50 to have the car taken to a wrecker's yard. It was more than a lemon by now. The engine needed extensive repairs, the gears were stripped, the suspension had collapsed, the tyres needed replacing, the front passenger door could not be opened, windows were broken, the outer body work was pitted with dings, and the interior was slashed and scratched. Like all of Riley's possessions, which he methodically destroyed or lost, his car did no better.

Chapter 6

Music was always important in Riley's life. His tastes were broad, and although he favoured the head-banging music that was popular with his generation, he also was partial to the Canadian singer, Anne Murray.

"If she comes to Brisbane to do a concert, Mum, let's go to see her. She said her family is more important than her career, so she must be nice."

Whenever she came on the radio, we would say in unison, "We'll go to see her if she comes to Brisbane. She's a family lady." It was a pact Riley and I had.

Anne Murray still hasn't come to Brisbane. If she ever does, I will go to see her. For Riley.

Riley always indulged me in my musical tastes by listening to Barry Manilow and the Mills Brothers. The boy-group Bros was popular with young people at the time – Riley liked them, too – and I told him that I was a groovy dame because I not only liked Bros, but I had one of their tapes.

"I don't believe you," he challenged. "Show me!"

When I produced my Mills Bros tape, Riley went into the scripted apoplectic fit.

"You're pathetic, Mum. What are you? Path--et--ic!!!"

And in Barry Manilow's 'Copacabana': does he call her 'over', or does he call her 'Rover'? We debated this riddle endlessly. We never tired of the same old hackneyed banter. They are memories of shared, happy moments.

About Madonna, I said, "Doesn't he play soccer well?"

Riley replied, "No, Mum. That's Maradonna."

"Doesn't she sing?"

"No, *that's* Madonna."

"Didn't he get into trouble for taking drugs?"

"No, Mum. *That* was Maradonna."

"Who? The Singing Budgie? Don't tell me the Singing Budgie takes drugs!"

"No! Mum! The Singing Budgie is Minogue — Kylie Minogue! Even you should know that!"

"He's Spanish, isn't he? He comes from one of those exotic Latin countries, doesn't he?"

"NO! NO, Mum! You're on to Maradonna again!"

"I've got it! I know now! He's the one with the sexy bottom that they're always photographing!"

With arms flailing, and much gnashing of the teeth, he admonished me, "You are a worry! A dead set worry! You know what it is, don't you? It's old age, Mum. The mind goes first, then it's curtains! There's no hope for you, you know. The nursing home won't know what hit them when you arrive. Here comes Mum! Watch out! Boy, do I feel sorry for them!"

We could never drive past a nursing home without his soliciting my opinion about its suitability as an abode for me in the near future.

"This one will be handy, Mum," he'd tease. "What do you think? It's close to home. I could walk down to visit you."

"I have no intention of going into a nursing home, Ril. It is my ambition to be a cranky and eccentric old biddy and live with you so that I can annoy you."

I reminded him of the bumper sticker that said: TAKE REVENGE. LIVE LONG ENOUGH TO BE A NUISANCE TO YOUR CHILDREN. "You have an obligation to care for me when I'm old. If it's on car bumper stickers, then it's a worldwide message. It's cast in stone. Every ageing mother in the world has the right to annoy her son. It's a universal law."

He laughed and said, "As if, sniff, Mum." One of Riley's favourite responses.

But just as Riley found joy in music, so too could he use it to punish himself. There was a tape that he had long desired, so I bought it for him. The following day, I found it completely unravelled, metres of knotted tape. "Why, Riley?" I asked. He had no answer.

When he felt that the ebb of his life was low, he would seek solace in music. During the last two weeks of his life, he listened intently and quietly to his music. He did this alone, in a reflective mood. There was no exchange of light-hearted repartee.

Prior to this, perhaps three months before he died, Riley gave me a Michael Jackson tape, specifically for the song titled 'You are Not Alone'. When he gave it to me, he said, "Always keep this near you, Mum. It's important. Okay?" He gave me a hug. I knew that it was a message, something that he wanted to tell me about his death, but that was in the future and the future was something I didn't want to deal with. But with his death, 'You are Not Alone' was his silent message. We played it at his funeral, and I know that his message was that he would always be with me.

As a mother, I carry a sense of guilt because I feel that I failed Riley. Children should have mothers whose maternal purpose in life is to nurture and protect them until they have the ability and life-skills to be self-sufficient, but I didn't.

At Riley's funeral, we also played Cyndi Lauper's song, 'Time after Time' because Coby told us that it was one of Riley's favourites. I wasn't aware of the song prior to his death, but when I listened closely to the lyrics, I realised that they poignantly reflected what I had been trying to do for Riley for twenty-six years. The song has a line that says, 'If you fall, I will catch you'. The radio station that I listen to plays this song often, and I am torn between a compulsion to listen to it and turning it off because I cannot bear the pain of knowing that, despite my best efforts, I did not catch Riley. Nor did I succeed in challenging the systems that I thought should be providing support for Riley.

Kevin and I have no doubt that the music Riley listened to, everything from the macabre messages of heavy metal rock bands to the hauntingly beautiful lyrics of conservative ballads, gave Riley comfort in deciding his final decide. Many parents blame the satanic lyrics of extreme rock groups for having some influence on their child's decision to suicide, but if one listens closely to the lyrics of many gentle ballads, unhappiness and loss are romanticised, and death, often depicted in heroic terms, becomes an alluring option, something for troubled minds to contemplate. These desperate souls are 'Candles in the Wind'.

As well as the comfort that Riley drew from music, he also found a haven in humour. No matter how bad things got, Riley could always dig deep and come up with a joke. He had a natural style that was droll and laconic, and he always laughed at his own funnies with a husky chuckle. When a momentous event happens in the public domain, in true Aussie style, the jokes start circulating immediately. Riley was always up to the moment with the latest classic one-liners, most of which he claimed he invented. I'd say to him after he told me a joke, "Where did you hear that?"

And he would say, "I just made it up."

I often told him he should be a comedian, but he looked questioningly at me because Riley never saw life as being funny. Sadly, it seems that the most publicly acclaimed comedians are often tragic in private.

When Riley told a blue joke, he would pat me and say, "You won't get this one Mum, but Dad will explain it to you later."

I cherished his belief in my innocence.

Chapter 7

Most of the distressing things that Riley did could be attributed to his mental instability. They were not deliberate acts of defiance or malice but the results of the troubled mind that controlled him. However, it is not my intention to idealise Riley by implying that his only flaw was his mental illness. On the contrary, in his rational moments he could try my patience to the limit and he often incurred my wrath.

One time, he and I had enjoyed a lazy Sunday morning together, and decided to go somewhere pleasant for lunch.

"So long as we don't go to one of those plant nurseries that you're so fond of Mum," he warned.

I assured him that we could find somewhere to eat that didn't sell plants, and then took a shower. When I got out of the shower, I called to him that the bathroom was free. But he didn't respond. I assumed he was outside having a cigarette. 'Best check that I've got enough cash for lunch,' I thought. But all my spare change was gone. I was puzzled and started recalling my shopping expeditions over the last few days and doing money sums in my head, trying to account for my lack of dollars, all the while getting dressed for lunch. Riley still hadn't come in for his shower, so I went outside to fetch him. That was when I saw that my car wasn't in the carport. At first, I couldn't believe that it wasn't there. I walked around the empty carport flapping my outstretched arms, feeling for the car. 'It's got to be here. It's got to be here somewhere,' I told myself. I wondered if I had forgotten that I'd parked it on the street. No, it wasn't there either. Perhaps the handbrake had failed and it had rolled down the hill to the bottom of the street? I walked the length of the street to check. It took me some fifteen minutes to realise that the absent Riley, my missing car, and lack of cash were connected. At first I was stunned, and then I got angry.

I raged around the house in the following days, giving vent to my anger. "How could he do this to me? The little bugger! How dare he! Just wait 'til I get hold of him. Damn him!" But in between my ranting and raving, I stood for long periods at the front windows, looking longingly down our street, willing him to come home, watching for a loved face to appear.

A week later we received a desperate phone call from him in an outer Sydney suburb. The car was not driveable, he had no money, and he was in a distressed mental state. Over the years, we had become experts at rescuing Riley from far away places, and we quickly organised Riley's journey home by bus, and had the car put on a road transport. Within a few days we had Riley and my car home again, both secure but neither in good working order.

On his return, he told us that his initial, impulsive reason for taking the car was to use it to kill himself by driving off an embankment or into a tree, but his thought processes went astray and he found himself in a familiar situation: frightened, and a long way from home.

Another time, he phoned me, serious and mysterious.

"I've got a confession to make, Mum," he confided. "I know you'll be upset, but I want to be up front and open about this."

"I'm listening, son," I said as I took a deep breath and braced myself for his revelation. This was a new experience for me as Riley had never forewarned us of events in his life before; he simply did them first and we found out later.

"I'm an alcoholic, Mum," he declared.

This didn't shock me because I was well aware that he liked a drink, but as far as I knew, he rarely had the cash in his pocket to buy alcohol on a regular basis. At home, he was quite content to share one or two beers with his father. However, he did over-indulge on occasions.

One day I arrived home to an empty house and found that someone had been physically ill in the hallway and bathroom. The stench of vomit and alcohol permeated the house. No attempt had been made to clean up the mess and I knew that Riley was the guilty party. To tone down my anger, I decided that before I cleaned the floors and walls, I would go for a power walk to dissipate my fury. But as I passed the local playground, I spied Riley sitting forlornly and drunkenly on a swing.

I strode over, grabbed him by the scruff of the neck, and frogmarched him home. "You little bugger!" I ranted. "What do you think you are doing? That's our home and you've fouled it. You're a bloody menace. If you were a puppy, I'd rub your nose in it!" I hardly paused for breath as I verbally pounded him with all my pent up frustration.

Riley said nothing. He just stumbled along, trying to keep up with me at a pace much too fast for someone in his condition. A neighbour who witnessed this pantomime cheered from his patio. "Give it to him, Til! You tell him, love!" He draped himself over the patio rails and laughed at the passing parade. But I was not disposed to share his mirth.

When we got home, I stood over Riley as I supervised the clean-up. I continued to scold him. When he dared to speak, all he could say was, "But Mum...I feel sick."

"Good! I'm pleased to hear it! You've missed a bit over there!"

A year or so after Riley died, I needed some Bailey's Irish Crème for a dessert recipe. 'I've had a bottle of that in the cupboard for ages,' I thought. 'I've never even taken it out of its packaging.' I rummaged around in the back of the cupboard and found the gift-wrapped liqueur. But when I unwrapped and uncorked the bottle, it was empty. Riley! I had no doubt that Riley had consumed the contents at some time in the past, perhaps even when he was sick in the hallway, rewrapped the bottle, and put it back where he had found it. This time I could not summon any anger. But I did indulge in a little melancholy chuckle.

What did shock me about Riley's drinking was how he was funding it. Riley was hocking our property!

Once, Kevin unwittingly tried to help after Riley decided to sell one of his two ghetto blasters to get some cash. "I'll go with you, son. I'll make sure you get a good price from the pawnbroker. You don't want to get ripped off, do you?"

"Thanks Dad. Let's go." Riley's understanding of life was so simplistic, he gratefully accepted his father's offer of help, not realising what was about to be revealed.

"G'day, Riley. Back again so soon? What have you got for us today?" The counter assistant greeted Riley like an old friend.

Kevin was taken aback by this familiarity. "Do you know him? What do you mean, 'What has he got for you today?' What's he got for you on other days?"

"Uh oh!" Riley plunged his hands into his jeans pockets, and stepped backwards slowly. His face paled. He tried to be inconspicuous. Tried not to be there.

"Well?" Kevin insisted.

"Let's see." The assistant counted on his fingers. "There was the whipper snipper. The radio. A variety of tools. Some commemorative coins and medallions. We gave you the joggers back, didn't we, Riley? We don't take used footwear. What else, Riley? I can't remember the other things."

Kevin was speechless. Riley looked mortified. The counter assistant suddenly realised what had just transpired. He looked from Kevin to Riley, and back to Kevin. "Oh," was all he could say.

We had been none-the-wiser. We had reported several missing items as stolen property to the police and assumed that other items that we could not find had been misplaced, and that they would turn up sooner or later. We never imagined the truth — that our property was stock on the pawnbroker's shelves.

A deal was never negotiated for the ghetto blaster. It came home with a chastened Riley who had some explaining to do. And I don't really know if it was my good fortune or Riley's consideration that saved some other valued items from finding their way to the pawnshop.

I have always kept treasured possessions in a bottom drawer, and among these tangible memories is jewellery that Riley bought for me. He took pleasure in doing this but he had a limited income and little understanding of value, and the various pieces never cost him more than twenty dollars each. But they are priceless in value to me. I wore the earrings and necklace he bought me to his funeral, and I never take the ring he gave me as a gift off my finger. At Brisbane's Expo, Riley had a broach made for me in gold coloured wire, which spelt out my name. I pinned this to the shirt he was cremated in.

Kevin placed his favourite handkerchief in Riley's shirt pocket when we said our last goodbye. "Have you got a clean hanky, Ril?" Kevin always asked before they set off on an outing, so he made sure that Riley had a handkerchief on his last journey.

In with my treasures is a blue ANZAC Day badge. My birthday is close to ANZAC Day and Riley's birthday gift to me one year was this badge because he knew of my admiration for old soldiers. Although it is now faded, it still shines brightly for me.

Riley had stayed with Coby on the weekend prior to his death. During the week following Riley's visit, Coby searched unsuccessfully for her newly purchased trendy sunglasses but assumed that she had mislaid them. They were sparkly, shiny blue, the colour so irresistible to bowerbirds. After Riley's death, his possessions were returned to us, and there were Coby's sunglasses. Our little bowerbird had nicked his sister's sunnies the previous weekend!

"If he wanted them that much, he can have them," Coby said as she placed them in his coffin along with various tapes of his favourite music.

Chapter 8

During one of Riley's many disappearances, I received a phone call from a detective in northern New South Wales.

"Mrs Brasch, I have Riley Brasch here in the police station. Your son, I presume. He has presented, claiming that he has been bashed about the head with a rock."

I interrupted with questions about his injuries.

"No, he's not badly hurt. But can you tell me something about him, please?"

I told him about Riley's mental health and his conduct.

"Just as I thought," replied the detective, kindly. "I think he's found himself a long way from home, and he's very frightened. He knows that we'll either detain him here, or take him to hospital. He's clobbered himself so that he could get a safe place to stay. I'll try to get him to go home, but if he won't, my church has a support group for young people like Riley. I'll talk to Riley, make some phone calls, and get back to you."

He phoned back soon after, and told me that he was taking Riley to a property in the Tweed hinterland where, in exchange for helping out on the property, Riley would receive board and lodging. The detective gave me the name and address of the family and encouraged me to visit as soon as possible.

Kevin and I drove there the next day. Riley was adamant that he wanted to stay, and the family seemed like good people. In a twist of fate, his job was to drive a tractor up and down a paddock, making straight furrows, but I don't think these people were onion farmers.

During his time at the property, Coby was married, and Riley's host family arranged for his transport to Brisbane and saw to it that he had a dinner suit, shirt, and bow tie.

"What do you think, Mum?" he said as he emerged from his bedroom, dressed for the wedding. "I chose this just for you," he added, fingering his purple bow tie. His faced glowed with pride.

"You look handsome, Riley," I said.

Riley was to accompany me until his father's duties with the bride were done. As I walked down the aisle on Riley's arm, I had the impression that his chest was puffed out and his head was held high. But, after the wedding, he insisted on returning to the property.

He stayed there for a few more weeks before moving on, and spent some time in northern New South Wales with a newfound friend.

One night as we arrived home from an outing, our car headlights picked out Riley standing on our driveway, head down and hands deep in his pockets. He was home once again. As usual, he was physically safe, but mentally fragile. He told us that his new friend had stolen a car and forced Riley to drive it while he held up a corner store, using a blood-filled syringe. Riley said he too had been threatened with the syringe. Perhaps this happened. Perhaps it didn't. But Riley wasn't smart enough to outwit the police, and as there was no inquiry by the law, nor any news items about such an event, I think it was another one of Riley's delusions. We could never be certain.

The police came to our home on another occasion to question Riley about his part in the theft of some racing saddles. The investigating detective seemed to understand Riley's mental incapacity and had a chat with Kevin and me about mental illness. Eventually he said, "As far as the theft goes, I'm not really interested in your son. I just need to clarify a few things that don't add up. I've got the real thieves. The smart little buggers are out in the car. They'll be stewing because they know I've sussed them. They've set your lad up, used him as a patsy." We heard nothing more about the stolen saddles.

The granny flat attached to our home was a place of solitude for Riley, where he spent many hours smoking and listening to music. At one stage, we set it up so that he could live there with the independence he desired. Its proximity to us meant that we could keep an eye on him, but it was far enough removed from the house to allow him to decide his own decides.

But he used its privacy as a place to harm himself. One time, he locked himself in the flat and phoned 000 to tell them that this was a siege and he was going to kill himself. He had cut himself badly and blood was sprayed on the floor and walls. The police arrived — we were not home — and the compassionate officer who attended the scene told Kevin later that at first they tried to talk Riley into giving himself up. "He wouldn't come out. He was defiant. I could see all the blood and I knew it was imperative that we get him out as fast as possible. I didn't know if he was going to bleed to death. In desperation, I yelled at him to come out, as if he was a naughty boy, and out he came. Meek as you like. I was surprised. But it worked and we could get him off to hospital quickly to have his cuts treated."

Kevin had been contacted by the police, and he arrived home after Riley was taken to hospital. On this occasion, the police told Kevin which hospital Riley was taken to, but as usual, the hospital did not contact us. The officer chatted to Kevin for some time about the complications of mental illness and law enforcement. He understood. But before I arrived home, Kevin cleaned up the blood to spare me the distress of seeing it.

One Christmas Eve, Riley was at home with us. He was full of the joy of the festive season and happily participated with the family in the last minute frenzy of wrapping gifts. There appeared to be peace and good will within our home. Suddenly, I realised that he had been gone from the room for a period of time, and my search found him downstairs in the granny flat covered in blood. He stood there snarling at me, holding out his up-turned bloodied arms like a sacrificial offering. I remember spinning on the spot several times, unable to decide whether I should run upstairs to get help or attend to him instantly, as he was obviously badly hurt. I gasped and gabbled as I ran to raise the alarm. When we all returned half a minute later to where he had been, he was gone, but his spattered blood covered the floor and walls.

Initially, we searched throughout the house and yard, and then Kevin and a friend drove around the neighbourhood looking for him, while Coby and I kept a vigil at home, in case he returned, or there was a phone call from a hospital about his welfare.

My instincts told me that he would make his way to the nearby psychiatric hospital, as he often did. I phoned.

"Riley's cut himself badly and disappeared," I frantically told the person who answered the phone. "We've looked everywhere for him, but we can't find him. Is he at the hospital?"

"I'm sorry, Mrs Brasch, but we are unable to release any information about patients." This was not an unfamiliar response.

"But he's hurt. He needs attention. If he's not at the hospital, we'll have to contact the police. We can't find him. He needs help." I was shouting.

"As I said, Mrs Brasch, we must abide by the rules of privacy."

"This isn't about your bloody rules! It's about my son's life! Is he there or isn't he?"

"I can neither say that he is, or that he isn't here. Good evening, Mrs Brasch." She hung up.

I made the same call another four or five times throughout the night — all with the same response.

I phoned the police, but their advice was to 'wait and see.'

As the night wore on into early morning, I became increasingly distressed. When I rang the hospital again at around 3.00am, a staff member with whom I had not yet spoken took pity on me because it was Christmas. Riley had been admitted.

"We've sutured his cuts, and he is resting under observation in the closed ward. You can visit him later in the day, Mrs Brasch."

"Thank you," I replied. "Merry Christmas."

When daylight came, I went to the hospital, but was not permitted to give Riley any of his Christmas gifts, and my belt and handbag were removed before I was admitted to the ward through a secure system of locked doors.

There was no visible evidence of the festive season in the ward. Several staff sat at a raised console where patients could be observed, while closed circuit television relayed the movements of other patients. Some patients paced in the enclosed grassed area, but there was no sign of companionable groupings, just lone figures with heads down. I walked past open rooms where I saw patients curled up like foetuses on beds, sleeping the familiar drugged sleep.

I tried to jolly Riley about his gifts, but he was not interested. I left in tears. It was Christmas Day, my son was in a locked psychiatric ward, he had cut himself seriously, and he didn't want to see me.

A burly staff member, who was escorting me back through the security doors, suddenly asked "When are you going to give up on him?"

"What? What do you mean?" The question stunned me.

"He's stuffing up his life. And nothing's going to change that. You shouldn't let him stuff up yours as well. You've got to think of yourself. Get on with your life. You've got to stop trying to pick up the pieces. You're wasting your life." By the time he had finished this tirade, he was shouting at me.

For the moment, my anger stifled my disbelief. "He is my son," I shouted back at him.. "He will always be my son. I will never give up." I hurried away and burst into tears. As I walked to my car, I asked myself repeatedly, 'Did I hear right? Could I have misunderstood?' I replayed the scene and the comments over and over in my head. It had happened.

When I got home, I told Kevin what had transpired.

"Forget it, Til," he advised.

"Shouldn't we report him or something?" I asked.

"And what would that achieve? I'll tell you what will happen. It'll get down to the nitty gritty of 'I said this' and 'he said that'. If there's trouble, he'll deny it, of course. Is that what you want? Haven't we got enough to cope with now without looking for more strife? Don't waste another thought on him, Til. You know and I know that we'll never give up on Riley. And Riley knows it, too. That's all that matters."

I took his advice.

Chapter 9

It was while Riley was a public mental health patient that he first experienced romance. He was so eager to have a girlfriend that he fell in love with any female who looked in his direction. He yearned for the reciprocal love that marked the natural transition from boyhood to manhood.

"Mrs Brasch, you don't know me. My name's Julie. I'm a patient at the same hospital as Riley. He's given me an engagement ring. I'm very upset about it. I don't know why he's done that. But I don't want the ring. I don't want to be engaged to Riley. I've tried to give it back, but he won't take it. Will you please come and get it? And talk to him for me please? I don't know what he thinks he is doing. I haven't encouraged him. It's just ridiculous!"

Riley had known Julie for only a few weeks. She most likely was kind to him, or sat and patiently listened to him.

I took the ring back to the jewellers and told them exactly what had happened. It had cost Riley his entire pension and they kindly refunded his money.

I had a fantasy that because Riley was gentle, kind, and gave his love so generously, a kind and competent girl would love him, care for him, and provide him with some semblance of a normal relationship.

Unfortunately, Riley's life revolved around mental institutions where he formed associations with people who were enduring the same difficulties as he was. And to form a romantic union with someone who was similarly mentally ill only doubled the existing problems for both parties. Nonetheless, Riley was ever the romantic.

His most serious foray into romance occurred with a young woman who we had known for a few years because of her periodic presence in the same psychiatric hospitals as Riley. Within three days of renewing their acquaintance, they were both discharged from hospital, and moved into a flat together. To complicate matters further, Rose was five months pregnant to someone else, but while living with Riley, she suffered a miscarriage. Riley was caring and supportive of her during this sad period.

Rose was a meticulous housekeeper and scrupulously clean. I wished her well at converting Riley to similar standards. At no stage of his life had Riley ever taken any interest in his surroundings. At home, his bedroom was just a space that had a bed in it where he could sleep. As he got older, he used the bed less and less and would roam about the house at all hours of the night, drinking strong coffee and going outside for cigarettes. And rather than make his bed each day, he would sleep on top of the covers, dressed in his day clothes, even in winter. Unless I objected, he would wear the same clothes day and night for weeks. "I like the smell," he would tell me when I told him he needed a shower because he reeked of stale sweat and cigarette smoke. Then when he did take a shower, he would stay under it until the hot water ran cold unless I raged into the bathroom and turned off the water, ordering him, "Out! Now!"

And when his bedroom needed redecorating, I asked him for his preference in colours and ideas. He looked at me and smirked, "Unless you're prepared to paper the walls with *Playboy* pages, I'm not interested." I wondered how Rose would cope with all of this.

Rose was also obsessed with the weekly budget and produced several budgets a week that she endlessly discussed with me. But the next day, there might be amendments to the budget, or a new budget and another consultation. And Rose always had a list of things that I had to buy for Riley – she deemed that to be my responsibility – like rubber thongs which she insisted he wear in the shower in compliance with her standards of cleanliness.

"This is what I have to buy this week." She showed me a neatly itemised list and went through each item telling me why it had to be purchased and the comparison of prices she had made. "Our combined pensions are this much," she said, indicating the sum of their pensions, "and I've priced everything on the list, so after the rent is paid, we'll have some money left over. That will go towards the engagement ring we're saving for." Her careful budgeting did make the purchase of an engagement ring a reality.

When I asked Rose what she wanted for Christmas, I was presented with a detailed list and cut-out pictures from newspapers and magazines of items from which to choose. Nothing was left to chance.

Dress, green, size 14. $59.95
Handbag, brown. $35.50
Slippers, pink. $19.99
6 glasses for juice. $15.00
Make-up – I'll come with you to choose

I called in at their flat on my way home from work every day to check on Rose and Riley because I was constantly concerned for their welfare. I always took some groceries or fruit to help them out and I chatted with them about their day, hoping to defray any potential problems. But they still arrived at our home later in the evening or in the middle of the night because Rose thought she might be ill or was worried about an issue. She thought that we favoured Coby over Riley and needed to discuss this with us often. "You gave Coby an engagement party. When are you going to do the same for us?" she pressed me. She continued, "My engagement ring is nicer than Coby's. I don't like hers. Mine is so beautiful. What do you think?"

"They're both lovely rings," I offered.

"Yes, but which one do you like best?" she demanded.

We often had this sort of discussion late at night after they had walked the three kilometres from their flat to our home. After an intense discussion, one of us then had to drive them home, dressed in our pyjamas. I became edgy, always waiting for that late-night knock at the door.

Rose watched me boil the jug to make a cup of tea one day. "Is that fresh water?" she asked.

"Fresh, about an hour ago," I told her.

"Tip it out and put fresh water in," she instructed. "I won't drink it otherwise."

Even today, if I reuse the water in the jug, my thoughts go to Rose.

"I'm sorry, Mum, but Rose needs to go to the doctor's again. Can you drive her please? She's too ill to walk." Riley made this request often but he was always apologetic because even he knew that her demands were excessive. Her illnesses were assorted: vague pains, earache, headache, a cold. "I just don't feel very well," she constantly complained. I spent many hours sitting in twenty-four-hour medical clinic waiting rooms.

Their relationship meant that Kevin and I spent a few months trying to support and guide not one, but two mentally ill people. Months passed and Rose's demands increased. Riley was embarrassed and apologetic but he thought it was his duty as Rose's partner to meet her needs.

I became so desperate to find a solution about how best to handle Rose, I consulted a doctor at the mental health unit they were both attending as outpatients and expressed my frustration at never seeming to meet Rose's needs. "You're wasting your time," the doctor informed me. "No amount of love, care, and attention will meet Rose's needs. No matter how much you give, she will demand more. She will emotionally exhaust you."

Rose desperately wanted to be a housewife and have a baby, but the thought of her and Riley as parents filled me with desperate fear. I knew that if they did produce a child, it would fall to Kevin and me to be the primary carers of this innocent baby. How could Riley and Rose take responsibility for an infant when they could not care for themselves?

"If I'm not pregnant this month, I'm going to make Riley go for a fertility test," she informed me several times. Fortunately for all concerned, a pregnancy did not result from their union before Riley opted to end the relationship. He too found Rose's demands physically and emotionally exhausting. We received another phone call. "Get me out of here, Dad. She's driving me crazy. I can't stand it another minute. Please come and get me."

"I'm on the way, son."

We were concerned about Rose's welfare, but she was philosophical about the end of their relationship. She even helped Riley and Kevin pack up his possessions. And, unexpectedly, she returned her beloved engagement ring to Riley, which he gave to me for safekeeping. However, following his death, I tried hard to trace her so that I could return the ring. I know how beautiful she thought it was and I wanted her to have it. But, despite searches in the phone book and more recently on the Internet, I have been unable to locate her. I still watch out for Rose in the faces that I see in crowded shopping malls. In her own well-intentioned but damaged way, she did try hard to create a normal relationship with Riley. She almost fulfilled my fantasy.

Soon after Riley's relationship with Rose ended, he found accommodation in a run-down boarding house, where Eddie also lived. They quickly became friends.

Eddie's clear complexion was the colour of milky coffee and he had dark, sparkling eyes. He was short and always neatly dressed. I never saw him in jeans or T-shirts. His youthful appearance belied a worldly-wise maturity.

Eddie always prompted Riley to be well mannered and considerate. "Help your mother out of the car, Riley." Or, "Have you offered your mother coffee?"

Eddie always asked about my day, and listened closely to every word I said. He was a suave and charming young man, with polished manners, and he came to our home on several occasions.

But soon after the friendship was formed, Riley asked me to hand over his life savings to Eddie. All of Riley's money was in a bank account, controlled by me. He wanted to give every cent he had to Eddie, who claimed that unless he paid the Australian government $4000 forthwith, he would be deported to India. It was strange that $4000 was exactly the amount in Riley's bank account.

"Eddie, Kevin and I are sorry to hear that you'll be deported if you don't pay $4000 to the government immediately, but I fail to see how it is our responsibility to rescue you."

"Just give him the money, Mum. It's my money and I want Eddie to have it. He's my friend and I want to help him," Riley instructed.

"What I would like Eddie to do first, Riley, is tell me how he plans to repay this money. It seems to me that if Eddie has the means to repay the money to us, then he has the means to meet the government's demand in the first place. If he's going to make repayments, then he can do that directly to the government. We don't need to be involved. What do you think, Eddie?"

"Well, if you could just see me out of this emergency, Mrs Brasch. It's a bit complicated, dealing with the government. I give you my word that you'll have the money back." As always, Eddie was smooth and smiling.

"Tell you what we'll do, Eddie. Kevin will help you draft submissions or letters to whoever it is in the government that is demanding this money from you, to plead your case. And then he'll set up appointments for you with the relevant departments. He'll even go with you, if you like, so that you can make personal representation about your deportation. If money is the key to your status here in Australia, perhaps some payment scheme that you can manage can be organised with the government. I think that's a reasonable compromise, don't you?"

"That's not what Riley wants," Eddie said, struggling to remain calm. "It is his money. And he wants to help me."

"We'll help you in any other way that we can," I assured him, "except giving you Riley's hard-saved cash. There will be no money changing hands. You can be certain of that. You do understand, don't you, Eddie?" I was intractable.

Riley was angry with me and Eddie continued to negotiate.

When Eddie accepted that no money would change hands, he disappeared, but not before we received a desperate phone call from Riley in the dead of night.

"Dad! Dad! Come and get me! You've got to come. Now! Please come and get me, Dad. Hurry, Dad!"

When Kevin arrived at the boarding house, Riley's room had been trashed. Personal items were smashed, including family photos. Riley was incoherent with fear.

"Where are his things?" I asked Kevin when they arrived home.

"There's nothing worth saving, Til, and unless you want to wash someone else's shit out of all his clothing, I didn't bring that home either."

Riley arrived home in just the clothes he was wearing. We were no longer shocked at these homecomings, just weary of the repetition.

In subsequent months, I arrived home from work one afternoon to find Riley and his latest friend, a stranger to Kevin and me, watching television in the lounge room. Peter had made himself at home, and was reluctant to leave when the evening got late. It was his intention to stay the night, but I ordered him out of the house. After our experience with Eddie, and other dubious people that Riley mixed with, I was suspicious of anyone who befriended Riley. Peter left that night, but he kept turning up at our home in the following days, and he soon endeared himself to us. Eventually, he took up our offer of accommodation in our granny flat where he lived for a few months.

Kevin and I came home late one evening to find a note on the table penned by Peter:

> *Have taken Riley to hospital. Don't think his leg is broken. Don't worry about the stove. I will pay for repairs.*

The stove? The stove! The oven door was kicked in. Peter had thought it might be useful to teach Riley some self-defence moves in the kitchen but with Riley's lack of coordination, the stove became an unintended target.

Peter had been a street kid, was street-wise, and had an indefatigable sense of survival. He seemed to attach himself to an array of people whom he claimed as relatives, but in reality, I believe they were just people whom he met as he passed through life. By 'claiming' them, he found the family that he desired. He called Kevin 'Dad' and me 'Mum'.

He was also an honest, loyal friend who mostly had Riley's best interests at heart. He was a decent young man. His childhood had been traumatic, but a cheeky grin, bubbly personality, and innate charm got him through life in spite of persistently difficult circumstances. He and Riley even looked alike with their blond curly hair and smallish stature.

Peter was convinced that he was a gift to every 'chicky babe' in Brisbane. He often came grocery shopping with us, and he maintained a constant commentary: "She's checking me out, Mum," or "Did you see that, Dad? She looked at me, eh, gave me the eye."

"Sorry mate, I missed that," Kevin responded. "I was too busy checking out the lovely Labrador she's got in that harness."

Peter told us that he couldn't read or write so I offered to teach him while he was with us, after I reminded him that he had written the note about the stove. Still, he insisted that he couldn't write. "You can do that for me, eh Mum, if I need something written down," he'd say when I urged him to write. But in the evenings after dinner, he would sit on the floor at my feet and read articles aloud out of the newspaper. He followed the words closely with his finger and only needed a little bit of prompting as he read slowly. Then he would beam the biggest smile when he got through the article. "You *can* read, Pete," I always told him.

"Well, the little words maybe, but not the big ones," he conceded.

Peter left us for a short period to work on a prawning trawler as a deck hand. "Can you swim, Pete?" I asked before he left.

"No," he said. "But sharks eat people who can swim, too, you know."

To take a lighter view of their relationship, Riley and Peter were Huckleberry Finn and Tom Sawyer incarnate. About a year into their friendship, both Riley and Peter disappeared without warning and we later discovered that because Peter disliked city life he decided he was going to live independently in the wild, off bush tucker. Peter told us many times: "The city sucks, eh? You'd be a mug to want to live in the city. Give me fresh air and wide-open spaces any day, eh. I can't cop streets and traffic and crowds and all that stuff."

Riley decided to join Peter on his outback odyssey. We were unaware that they had hitchhiked up the Queensland coast until we heard from a frightened and hungry Riley a few weeks later. They had reached the wilderness on the Cape York Peninsula, and were at a place called Lakefield, and, when Riley called again later, he was at Laura.

"I'm frightened, Dad," he said. "I'm too scared to sleep. There are things here that either want to bite me or eat me. I can't remember when I last had a meal. I want to come home, Dad. Can you get me home, please?" He sounded exhausted.

"What about Peter? Is he okay?" Kevin asked.

"Bugger Pete. He's happy here. He must be bloody mad to want to be with crocodiles and snakes and mosquitos. I just want to come home, Dad."

With our acquired skills, we were able to contact the local police and make arrangements for Riley to be picked up and taken to the nearest town that had an intrastate bus service, but only after Kevin had done verbal battle with the cynical young police constable who had no sympathy for Riley's situation until Kevin threatened to phone the Police Commissioner to inform him that Riley was at risk and assistance had been refused. Only then was Riley given overnight hostel accommodation, put on a bus the following day and returned to Brisbane.

We asked the police to check on Peter also, but we were assured that he was in his element, and quite content to stay where he was, for the time being, anyhow.

Immediately after Riley died, a friend tried to locate Peter to tell him about Riley's death, but he was such an itinerant character with the most common surname, the search was fruitless. Two years later, Peter was on our doorstep, cheeky grin still in tact.

"G'day, Dad. It's me, eh. I'm back. Rile home?"

"Peter, Riley died. We tried to find you, mate."

Peter giggled. "Yeah? Still cracking the jokes, eh, Dad? But that's a bit sick-o. Come on, where's Riley?"

"Come with me, Peter." Kevin took Peter to Riley's bedroom and got out the box of sympathy cards and other keepsakes. Peter slumped on to Riley's bed, crying, wringing his fists in his eyes like a little child. Kevin gently told him what had happened.

We asked him to stay, but he didn't want to. As he left the house, head low and shaking in disbelief, he was still crying. He kept repeating, "He's dead. He's dead."

We haven't seen Peter since that awful day, but maybe he will come back to us eventually.

In spite of his bad experience on that trek with Peter, the lure of North Queensland beckoned Riley once again. He was befriended by a man who was working some sort of credit card scam in the Townsville and Charters Towers regions. Riley phoned us. "You've got to get me out of here. This bloke makes me go into banks and get money with dodgy credit cards. I don't want to do it but he says he'll belt me if I don't. I'm frightened. Help me, Dad. You've got to help me."

Riley gave us an address that we were able to pass on to a dear friend who lived in Townsville.

Henry had represented Queensland as a rugby league front row forward, where only the toughest of the tough survive, and although he has a quiet and gentle nature, his sheer size and calm self-assurance ensures that things will be done his way. He is a man of few words, but steady eye contact, a half enigmatic grin, and a forward inclination of his huge frame gives an indisputable impression that he does not wish to be challenged. The body language says, 'Do not mess with me!'

Without hesitation, Henry went to the address, removed Riley, looked after him overnight, and saw him safely on to a bus the following day, which brought Riley back to Brisbane. Again.

Riley also had to make his way back from Melbourne once, where he had gone with a girl who had a pet rat. A thoughtful truck driver picked them up as hitchhikers and recognised that Riley needed help. The truckie brought him back to Brisbane. I don't know what happened to the girl or the rat.

"Where's your gear, Riley?" I asked him on his return. He had nothing with him, just the clothes he was wearing. He looked haggard.

"In Melbourne, I think. I'm not sure. I don't remember. I just had to get out of there, Mum. They were weird people."

"What people, Riley?"

"I don't know. There were people there. I don't know who they were. But I was frightened." He was home again.

When Riley wasn't fraternising with his assortment of mates and girlfriends, I tried to have an outing with him at least once a week. But they weren't always pleasant occasions.

Riley and I were going to the movies, but first we were going to have dinner at a large fast food restaurant. We had ordered our meal, but while waiting for it to be served, Riley's mood changed suddenly. Until this moment, everything was pleasant and normal.

Nothing had happened to cause Riley distress. It was as if a switch had been thrown.

His heavy breath came through clenched teeth and his eyes glowered. His glare came at me from under his brows.

"What am I doing here with you? Why do I have to be with you?" Hate was in his eyes.

I put my arms around the table accoutrements. I sensed that he was about to clear the table with one swipe. "We're going to have dinner and then we'll go to the movies, Riley. I thought you were looking forward to tonight. You've picked the movie. Let's enjoy ourselves." I tried to sound calm and nonchalant. "They should bring our meal soon."

"Stuff the bloody meal! I'm outa here!" He shoved the table at me as he tried to stand.

I put my hand on his arm. "Wait, Riley. Just sit down, son. I can't leave now. And I can't let you go on your own. We've ordered a meal and I haven't paid for it. We'll be in strife if we just walk out. And I don't want to pay for a meal that I haven't eaten. Come on. Let's just sit quietly for a while." I could feel the tears welling.

With another hefty shove of the table and his chair falling over backwards, he stormed towards the centre of the restaurant. I couldn't distinguish the words of his verbal explosion. People looked up, startled.

I rushed after him and tried to physically restrain him. In front of a large crowd we had a sort of passive wrestle. I was crying. Riley was having quite a bit to say, but no one came to my aid, and nor did anyone ask if I was okay. All eyes were turned away and people continued to eat their meals as if Riley and I were invisible. I was more devastated by the reaction of the other diners than I was by Riley's behaviour.

I don't remember paying the bill. Maybe I did. Maybe I didn't. I think the staff were pleased to have Riley and me off the premises at any cost. We didn't see the movie either.

There were many movies that Riley and I did see together and enjoyed in a companionable way, but he was always unpredictable:

"We're going to the movies, Riley. Do you want to come with us?" I asked.

"No, I don't want to go," he responded.

"Okay. We'll be leaving as soon as we're ready."

"That's right, leave me at home," he hissed. "Don't bother about me. You run off and see your movie."

"I've asked you to come with us, son. I'd like you to come with us. What say you get dressed and come with us?" I cajoled.

He did, but refused to come into the theatre complex with us. He sat on the bonnet of our car, in the car park, for the duration of the movie. When we emerged after the movie, Riley was seething. "Enjoy your movie? Yeah, I bet you did. Just run off and leave me. You don't give a stuff, do you?" We called this Riley's 'Yes, No' game and no matter how hard we tried to decipher his mixed messages, it was always confusing. He said 'Yes' when he meant 'No', and 'No' when he meant 'Yes', and just when we thought we had made a correct interpretation, 'Yes' meant 'Yes', and 'No' meant 'No'. Sometimes. Most of the time. Or not at all. Simple communication was habitually bewildering and complex.

Chapter 10

For the duration of Riley's illness, we were given advice by friends and acquaintances about how we should deal with him. It covered every aspect of treatment and behaviour modification, ranging from alternative medicine, what the friend of a friend did, to disowning Riley: 'If he was my son, I wouldn't stand for that sort of nonsense. Don't let him back in the house until he can behave. You haven't got to put up with that.'

Advice from others usually implied that they knew better than we did about coping with mental illness. Negotiating this advice became so problematic we ceased discussing Riley's illness with most people. It was easier not to deal with other's misconceptions about our reality. Our reality was that Riley's daily life mostly resembled a disjointed nightmare that had no rhyme or reason: fragments of behaviour and events peppered us like swirling grains of sand in a sandstorm. But even when Kevin and I had our daily discussions about incidents concerning Riley, we found that we automatically converted them into our version of a 'normal', rational context and we applied our logic, which, in fact, misrepresented what Riley actually did.

A wet towel on the bathroom floor could lead to a typical, but incomprehensible exchange.

"Riley, can you hang up your bath towel, please?" What mother hasn't made this request?

"That's right, say it was me!" he responded with malice.

"Well, this is my towel, and that's your father's. So this wet one on the floor must be yours." The logic seemed simple to me.

"Well, I won't go. You can forget it!" His logic.

"Go where?" I inquired.

"Why don't you just call me a dick-head!"

"I'm not calling you anything, son. I just want the towel hung up. It's easy."

"And you can forget about dinner. I don't want your bloody food. Why don't you run off and talk to your precious daughter." Spite was never an element of Riley's character but he sometimes resorted to this sort of comment as the ultimate barb.

"Hold on. Just take a deep breath, Riley. This is about your towel. Nothing else. Nobody else. And what has food got to do with picking up your bath towel?" I knew this was a redundant question, but I had to ask if only to try to make sense of it all to myself. "It would be so easy just to hang up your towel, Ril."

He stood there defiantly, glaring hatred at me, breathing heavily through clenched teeth. The towel remained on the floor and he didn't eat with us. He stormed out of the house after punching a few walls on the way out. "I've broken my knuckles now. Satisfied?" he spat at me. After an episode like this, it could be a week before we saw him again, or we might get a phone call from a hospital telling us he had harmed himself and was in intensive care. Maybe it was after this altercation that he overdosed on Panadol.

"He's lucky to be alive, you must realise. This is the largest overdose of paracetamol we've ever had in this Intensive Care unit. Others who have taken much less have not survived," counselled the young doctor on duty in the intensive care ward that Easter weekend. "But he's not out of the woods yet, mind you. That amount of Panadol will damage his liver. We'll just have to wait and see how he comes out of this. Only time will tell how much damage he's done."

But there was no liver damage. He had overdosed twice before and again, inexplicably, he had defied the odds.

His sense of devilment wasn't damaged either. He was the only patient in the IC ward and as far as he was concerned, boredom was his greatest affliction. Reclining in the intensive care capsule and hooked up to various monitors, he said, "Watch this." He proceeded to over-breathe, sort of hyperventilate, and the machines started buzzing and ringing urgently. All those zig-zaggy lines on the screens went haywire. The nurse came running and was not amused. "Riley, I've told you not to do that! It's not funny! Don't do it again!"

"Well, I'm the only one here and if I don't keep you on your toes, you'll be as bored as I am. We can't have that, mate," Riley offered by way of appeasement.

With the passing of the years, Riley's illness began to take its toll on me. I came to a slow, demoralising realisation that all my efforts amounted to a consistent record of failure with not one encouraging success to give me heart or the energy that I needed to face the future. I was mentally and physically exhausted. I was defeated. Only with hindsight do I now recognise my own downward spiral into a state where I was barely coping, certainly not with Riley, and only just hanging onto the threads of my own sanity. I did silly things like putting the sugar in the fridge and I got into the shower a few times with my glasses on. I'd forget to turn the stove on when I cooked a meal. I'd stand at the stove wondering why the pot didn't boil. But on other occasions, I'd forget a saucepan on the stove, and only remember it when the smell of burning food filled the house. I seemed to be in a domestic vortex.

More seriously, I remember being concerned about my driving performance. I often rebuked myself: 'You've got to get your act together or you'll have to stop driving, my girl. This is not good. You're a danger to yourself and others.' My mind was so addled, I couldn't make sense of the movement of traffic around me on the road. Cars seemed to come at me from all directions causing me to panic and take the wrong option. On a few occasions, I stopped at the green traffic lights and was alarmed that other cars continued to drive through the intersection. 'What are they doing? They should be stopping!' It was only when horns tooted behind me that I realised the light was green and I should not have stopped. Red lights caused me a problem too. A few times I came to a shuddering, sudden halt at the last moment, brakes screeching and tyres burning rubber. Fortunately, my fellow motorists and I survived this period of mental lapse, but I was regularly the recipient of verbal abuse and much horn honking.

It was about this time that I realised I needed to do something positive for myself to distract me from the increasing intensity of

Riley's turmoil and the toll his dysfunctional behaviour was having on me. A friend who understood gave me an Eileen Caddy poster that said:

YOU ARE NEVER ASKED TO DO MORE THAN YOU ARE ABLE
WITHOUT BEING GIVEN THE STRENGTH AND ABILITY TO DO IT.

I stuck it up on the wall of my office and read it whenever I needed to find reserves of emotional strength. I knew that I had to stay strong not only physically, but also emotionally. If I became ill, what would happen to Riley? I instinctively knew that I had to find something to focus on, something just for me, something that had nothing to do with Riley's daily chaos.

Finally, I decided to undertake a Bachelor of Arts degree. For a few hours of each week, I steeled myself to void my mind of all matters other than the academic content of lectures and tutorials, and I believe that this helped keep me sane.

But still, the pull of Riley's influence was difficult to resist.

In preparation for one particular final exam, I purchased a new pencil case a few weeks before the exam date, and filled it with the essentials: writing materials, I.D. card, tissues, and mints, and then put it away securely so that, on the day, I was all prepared to go. No fuss. No bother. Organised.

Fancy that, I thought, when I saw a similar pencil case on Riley's desk – he was living at home at this time. That's the same as my new pencil case. I guess they're popular in the shops at the moment. But as Riley had a penchant for bringing things home that no amount of cross-examination would reveal the origins of, I gave it no further consideration. He continued to be a bowerbird, right up until the end.

For a day or two, the situation didn't bother me. But eventually, something niggled at me, and I checked out his new pencil case.

"Riley, this is my pencil case! What are you doing with it? Bloody hell! Can't you see that it's all set up for uni and my exam? Is nothing safe around here?"

"Oh…yours, is it? Well, there you go. Settle down, Mum. Keep your hair on. You've got it back now. What's the problem?"

"Just keep your sticky fingers off my things. Leave my things alone. Is that clear?"

But more was to come of this. On the day of the exam, I was about to set off for the university, pencil case in hand when Riley stopped me.

"Social Security needs a letter from you about where I am living," he announced.

"I'll do it when I come home, Riley."

"No, Mum. They need it this morning. By ten o'clock. Otherwise I lose my benefits."

"You're joking! When did they tell you this, Riley?"

"A few weeks ago. I just remembered now."

I was fuming. So much for planning my time.

"I can't do it now, Riley. I'm late already."

"No, Mum," Riley said, pursuing me out to the car. "This is my last chance. You've got to do it now!"

"You're the one who's messed up, so you'll have to suffer the consequences. I've got an exam to do! Thanks a lot, Riley. This is just what I don't need!" I backed out in a rage.

By the time I arrived at the university, my anger had abated and I decided to write the letter for him. This necessitated buying suitable paper and envelope from the university bookshop, composing the relevant details, and scratching around for correct change to phone a taxi to meet me at an appointed place so that the document could be couriered to the Social Security office. As I waited for the taxi, I could see my fellow students filing into the Great Hall, but still the taxi had not arrived. My brain was in turmoil. I could almost taste my panic. Hurry, hurry, I silently willed the taxi.

Eventually the taxi arrived, just as I saw the doors of the Great Hall close, marking the start of the exam.

"Hello, love. You phone for a delivery? What's the job?" a kindly driver asked, as he alighted from the cab. He had no urgency in his manner.

"This envelope. To this address. Before ten o'clock. It's urgent. How much?"

"Aw. Let's see. How far would that be?"

"Charge me for thirty kilometres. How much?"

"No. Let's get this right. I'll radio base...."

"No. Please. I'm in an awful hurry. My exam has started."

"Base? St Lucia to Chermside? How far is that? Twenty-five clicks? Thanks, Steve. No, I'm at the university now. Yup, I've found the lady."

"How much?" My eyes constantly flicked in the direction of the Great Hall.

"Let's say forty dollars will cover it, love. Fair enough? You don't want to be paying for more miles than it is. Can't throw money away, you know. Too hard to come by. Now, what's my best route? I'm not too familiar with the north side. If I get back to Hale Street, then what? Would I be best going via Gympie Road or Webster Road? What's my best option?" He was relaxed, ready for a chat. I was tense, ready to run.

"Gympie Road. Gympie Road's the most direct route." I held the money out to him. I didn't want to offend him with my haste because I needed his cooperation.

"What about parking? Is parking available? No good if I can't park. Sometime I have to drive round and round to find where I can park. Jolly waste of time for everyone."

"Gympie Road. Turn right at Banfield Street. Park underneath. It's easy. Here. Forty dollars. It's got to be there before ten o'clock. Thanks." I had already taken a few steps towards the Great Hall.

"Thanks, love. You have a nice day now."

Over my shoulder as I increased my speed towards the Great Hall, I called back to him, "Yes. You too. Thanks."

A frantic run got me to the Great Hall fifteen minutes late to start the exam, but my mind was not in exam mode. It occurred to me that chaos was my constant, unwelcome companion. Nonetheless, Riley retained his social security benefits and I passed the exam.

On another occasion, a week before I had an exam to sit, Kevin and I spent that time searching for Riley after he had disappeared from home. Eventually, on the evening before the exam, we traced him to the Salvation Army Hostel for Homeless Men at Spring Hill where he had been living for the week. While Kevin was inside the hostel getting Riley's effects together and paying for his accommodation, I sat outside in the car, trying to study by the interior cabin light.

In the last two years of Riley's life, I mostly went with the flow of his disorder. I dealt with events in a resigned manner after they had occurred rather than trying to prevent them, as I had done for many years. All the fight in me was spent. What I thought was a bottomless well of determination to make Riley's life safe, comfortable and worthwhile did in fact have a bottom, and I had hit it hard. My repetitious efforts to scale the slimy black walls of this dark and murky well constantly sent me plummeting back to the bottom. For me, the last six months of Riley's life passed as if I was observing it through a fuzzy haze. I was mostly unaware of what was happening around me. I couldn't think things through, and the simplest of tasks seemed like the tallest of mountains that I had to climb with a weary body and fatigued mind.

Chapter 11

We didn't know it at the time, but Riley's brief ownership of the car, in part, inadvertently took him to the next stage of his life. He was charged with the following offences:

Defendant's Criminal History

1. Possession of a dangerous drug (cannabis sativa) on 4th September 1992;

2. Unlawful possession of a pipe used in connection with smoking the drug;

3. Possession of a .22 rifle whilst not holding the relevant licence under the Weapons Act 1990.

4. On 1st February 1993, possession of a pipe for the purpose of smoking a dangerous drug;

5. On 2nd June 1993, breach of a community service order;

6. In July 1992 breach for failure to wear a seat belt;

7. In April 1992, driving whilst holding a provisional licence with a BAC of .027.

When we read the charge sheet, we were alarmed. We knew of Riley's marijuana usage and his occasional alcohol excesses, but it was his possession of a gun that shocked us. Riley had never shown an interest in guns and no one in our family, nor anyone in our circle of friends, had any interest in guns.

"What were you doing with a gun, Rile?" we asked.

"It's not mine. It's Luke's. He said my car would be a good place to store it. I told the copper it wasn't mine, but he said that's what they all say. I was just minding it, Mum."

Riley had been stopped for a roadside breathalyser test, and the unconcealed gun was spotted on the back seat of his car. Riley had been in the courts before for marijuana possession and legal advice was that on this occasion, he may have to serve a jail sentence because not only were the charges more serious, but he had reoffended.

As a result of the charges brought against him, Riley was directed to present himself for interview at a suburban police station. As I drove him there, I raged: "What the bloody hell do you think you are doing? You know damn well that this is not acceptable behaviour. You've committed crimes! The police will deal with you now. Let's see how you handle that, you smart little bugger! And you want to muck about with drugs, do you? Well, let's see what the police think about that. You're not dealing with your parents now, you know. You've got to face the law and the law won't take any of your nonsense." I all but shoved him out of the car door when we arrived at the police station. "Now get in there and take your punishment!" I let him go into the police station alone while I sat in the car park fuming, waiting for Riley to emerge after his interview. And all the way home, I kept up a tirade about his behaviour.

Since Riley was twelve years old, medical advice consistently had been that his problems were behavioural, and, because a mental illness was not diagnosed, I foolishly believed that he should face up to the consequences of his behaviour as a normal member of society.

I thought that intervention by the law would make Riley realise that dabbling in drugs and his other misdemeanours would not be tolerated and that these things had legal consequences. It was my hope that he would 'get his act together and smarten up' as advised by the psychologist who called him a bastard.

However, through the rest of the day, I thought of little else but our visit to the police station and my anger. Something was bothering me and I couldn't shake it off. As I was preparing the evening meal, after my anger had abated, it occurred to me that I was uncomfortable because I knew that I was wrong. My scepticism about the bad behaviour theories had been increasing in recent times, and I was becoming more and more conscious that the normal world was not Riley's world. Riley was not in touch with reality and we were out of our depth in dealing with his problems. I had treated Riley harshly at the police station and allowed my anger — and fear — to overshadow a compassionate perspective. Following this particular police interview, I became resolute in my determination that the law should not punish Riley for the tragic hand that genetics had dealt him. Riley needed my love and support, not my wrath and rejection.

His conduct was not bad behaviour, but something far more serious. We had always struggled to accept the bad behaviour theory because it was contrary to our gut feelings, but as had been the case when Riley was an infant, we trusted that the medical profession knew better than we did, especially when dealing with the complexities of psychiatrics.

After discussing my feelings with Kevin, we contacted a barrister friend who advised us that, legally, Riley had not been obliged to make himself available for interview, and if he had, he should have had legal representation. Obviously, the police knew these points of law, but didn't inform us of Riley's legal rights. And all that would have been beyond Riley's comprehension. The charges proceeded to a Court appearance.

When we consulted our legal friend about the charges, we were advised to have a psychiatric assessment done on Riley's mental health to present to the Court. Consequently, Dr Cooper entered our lives. He prepared a report that was tendered to the magistrate in 1993 to plead the case against the possibility of Riley serving a jail term. The report was successful and saved him from going to jail. Instead, Riley received a community service order and fine.

To start with, Dr Cooper's report stated that he would conduct a series of assessments and interviews, as well as accessing records of Riley's previous psychiatric treatment.

The report continued:

> *Riley is a seriously damaged/demolished personality, because his intelligence is at the bottom of the population ladder and at the top of the mentally retarded ladder;*
>
> *This led to brutal rejection at an academic private school during secondary studies;*
>
> *Psychiatric assessments over the years apparently were incomplete and he was dealt with superficially leading to repeated rejection by helpers;*
>
> *This professional stance misled the family to take a punitive ("you're not measuring up") approach in trying to help Riley;*

> *His anger, frustration and suffering have been expressed by suicide attempts, self-mutilation (symbolizing being torn-apart by performance demands he could not meet) acting-out behaviours crying for help and attention;*
>
> *Superficial and inadequate therapeutic responses have obscured his courage and grit in staying alive and repeatedly "picking himself-up, dusting-off and starting all over". - the story of his life since the bastardizing began at St Jude's School at age 13;*
>
> *He is a product of failed psychiatry.*

Dr Cooper's report also acknowledged Riley's 'commitment to and love of his family', and added that it was fundamental to Riley's rehabilitation that he not be burdened with the public label of "border-line mentally retarded" because "he has abilities which are still obscured and distorted by his disturbances".

At last, a decade after we first sought medical help for Riley's behaviour, we had something that enlightened us to the complexities and seriousness of his illness and we were encouraged that the doctor also rejected the bad behaviour theories. But still, we were not given an actual diagnosis.

During the last decade, many psychiatric illnesses had been mentioned, but none were confirmed: Issues with anger? Troubled teenager? Attention seeking? Manic depressive? Behavioural disorder? Bipolar disorder? Once, I accidentally overheard one of the nursing staff use the word 'psychotic' in relation to Riley.

"Is he psychotic? No one has ever used that word before. What does it mean? Is that what we are dealing with? What can we do about it?"

"We're not sure," she replied. "I don't think so, but it's not for me to say."

"Well, who can tell me?" But there was never an answer.

I asked his primary care nurse if Riley was schizophrenic. "No, he's not schizophrenic, although his symptoms do mirror schizophrenia," she replied. "We don't believe he is hearing voices. We suspect he is imitating the behaviour of schizophrenic patients he observes in hospital."

By this time, we had discovered that unless our friends and acquaintances received a specific answer to their questions about what was wrong with Riley so that they could label or categorise him, they had trouble understanding the nature of his illness. The reasoning seemed to be that if he was ill, then the illness must have a name. People like labels so that they can slot things into familiar areas of knowledge for which they have reference points, but Riley was in limbo when it came to putting a name to his illness. Yes, it was a mental illness, but what sort of mental illness? I often lamented, 'If only his illness had a name, we would reduce our problems. But we can't begin to make things right if we don't know what's wrong.'

Our initial purpose in contacting Dr Cooper was to obtain the psychiatric report for Riley's Court appearance, but we were also advised to place Riley in this doctor's care because he was held in the highest regard by Brisbane's legal fraternity: "When mentally ill people run foul of the law, this guy is as good as having God in your corner," was our legal advisor's opinion of Dr Cooper.

On our first visit to the doctor's dimly lit rooms, we waited an hour or more for our appointment. We soon discovered that the doctor was never on time for the appointments that we had with him. His waiting room was tired-looking, and out-of-date magazines cluttered what space was not occupied by waiting patients. Some patients stood in the corridor for want of seats. As we waited, my gaze kept going to the crooked painting on the wall that I had an urge to straighten. When we were ushered into his consulting room, we sat at a low, round table, which occupied a small space among other pieces of furniture, all cluttered by files, equipment, and books.

Dr Cooper was a big man who seemed to carry a heavy weight on his broad, drooping shoulders. He always seemed to be harried and careworn, and he often appeared in the media as the expert psychiatric witness in serious criminal trials.

Dr Cooper's initial priority was to evaluate Riley's mental condition and establish a treatment and medication regime, which we assumed would put Riley on the road to management of his illness, if not a recovery. To commence treatment, Dr Cooper admitted Riley to the acute psychiatric section of Keswick Private Hospital, initially for a period of two weeks. However, it was three years and seven months before Riley was discharged.

Not long after Dr Cooper admitted Riley to Keswick, I realised that this weary man was over-committed and there were never enough hours in the day for him. His visits to Riley were often late at night. Still, he was a constant strength in Riley's treatment.

Although Riley never remarked, I had a sense that he was fond of Dr Cooper. Even so, they had a dynamic relationship and Riley often verbally abused and sacked the doctor.

When I asked Doctor Cooper why he continued to treat Riley after these episodes, he laughed. "That sort of stuff goes with the territory. I don't take any notice." He waved his hand dismissively. "Anyhow, I doubt if Riley will remember that he has sacked me when next we meet. I'm sure I've still got a job." He was always right.

Riley also kicked in Dr Cooper's car door in a fit of rage, but still the doctor forgave him. Riley paid to repair the damage, and the doctor continued to treat Riley until three months before he died, almost four years. Through it all we kept waiting for a miracle to happen. But there were never any miracles for Riley.

When we questioned how long Riley's treatment was taking, we were told that an assessment of his complex problems was progressing and that his medication had to be constantly adjusted to find what combination of drugs would control or alleviate his symptoms. "We need to see what works for him," the doctor advised, "and we need to keep him under observation to do this."

As Riley's stay in Keswick became more extended, we wanted him to come home, but because he was over eighteen we had no power to remove him from the hospital or put a stop to any of his medical treatments. And it was during his early days at Keswick that Dr Cooper arranged for Riley to appear before the Mental Health Tribunal when it was determined that he should be a regulated patient. In subsequent years, Riley was assessed by another two Patient Review Tribunals under the *Mental Health Act 1974* with the decisions being consistently that 'the Tribunal recommends that it is necessary in the interest of the patient's own welfare that he continue to be liable to be detained'.

This was in place during the last three-and-a-half years of

Riley's life and meant that his mental health was a fact at law, and although it did afford him some protection under the *Mental Health Act*, his regulation, plus his status as a legal adult removed us from all decision-making processes that related to him. Nor were we entitled to be informed about any aspect of Riley's life unless he gave permission.

Apart from medication, an early therapy was to find something to interest Riley, a positive replacement activity, like a fitness program at a gym. The philosophy was that if he could take pride in his body through regaining the fitness level of his earlier years, he would cease to abuse it. At best, Riley was erratic in attending the gym, and his interest soon petered out. But his self-harm continued. And it was during these early days at Keswick that his self-harm graduated to serious mutilations.

Riley was always inventive at finding ways to harm and punish himself. He even did substantial damage once by gouging himself with a thumbtack and he regularly damaged the hospital by breaking windows and smashing crockery to obtain sharp fragments with which to slash himself. He cut his forearms, chest, and legs so often, eventually the doctors were unable to suture the masses of keloid scarring.

On a few occasions, he boiled the jug and poured the boiling water over his left forearm. On a break away from the hospital, we took him to Hervey Bay one Easter, but the time was spent dressing severe burns from one of these events, and he couldn't swim nor go onto the beach because of his burns. And he heated the iron and placed it on his arms.

He cut his throat several times, requiring microsurgery and intensive care hospitalisation twice. After one of these incidents and surgery to repair his sub-jugular, the theatre staff at the large metropolitan hospital kindly allowed Kevin and me to go in to him in the recovery room. I found Riley on a trolley-bed, drips and monitors attached, covered to his neck in blankets, with his head wrapped in a blanket too, like he had been as a baby in the frail nursery with just his face showing. I put my arms around him as best I could and was speaking to him when Kevin came to my side.

"That's not Riley, Til. Rile's over there." I had been comforting the wrong person. I couldn't even recognise my own son, such was my wretchedness. Despair had blurred my vision.

But another incident while he was in Keswick is indelibly etched in my memory above the others. After cutting his throat in a park, he walked back to the hospital along a busy main road, covered in blood, but no one stopped to help him. He was so badly cut that he required surgery and intensive care hospitalisation once again. The nursing staff were stunned that he was able to make the walk without collapsing from loss of blood. His clothes were so stained with blood, they were thrown away, but a nurse gave me his joggers. "These are almost new," she said, handing me the blood-saturated joggers. "If you soak them in cold water and then give them a hard scrub, they'll come up as good as new. They're too good to throw out."

I soaked them in the laundry tub, and as I scrubbed them, I looked at the deeply bloodstained water in the tub, and realised that this was my son's blood, shed in an effort to take his life. My sobs choked me. I slumped over the tub, holding on tightly so that I didn't fall to the floor. It was in the flash of moments like this that the full reality of Riley's difficulties and our daily involvement in his mental health problems hit full force. Denial becomes reality. It's easy to think that you are coping, perhaps even essential to believe that you are coping so that some shred of sanity can be retained, but the fact is that we never fully coped.

Apart from venting his anger and frustration on Dr Cooper, Riley regularly absconded from Keswick. "Guess what?" Riley spoke in a confidential whisper with a conspiratorial smile on his face. "We escaped today."

"Who is 'we', and where did 'we' escape from?" I asked. I had just arrived in the hospital's secure courtyard to visit Riley.

"Me, Michelle, Jenny, Mike, Davo. Some of the others wanted to come, but they're not fit enough. They would've slowed us down, so we had to leave them behind. If you stand right back here and take a running jump onto that table, it's easy to make it to the top of the wall. Then all you have to do is drop into the garden on the other side. How easy is that? Then it was every man for himself. I was off down the hill with the speed of a thousand green ants!"

Jack Nicholson in *One Flew Over the Cuckoo's Nest* came to mind.

Riley escaped from the hospital regularly but he hadn't taken others with him before. From his presence, though, I guessed that he and his mates hadn't got far before the fugitives were rounded up. Riley's escapes meant that the local police had the repetitive task of returning him to the hospital. "How far did you get today, Riley?" I would ask after learning that once again, he had 'done a runner', as he would say.

"Just down the road."

"How come you're back then?" I asked.

"It's the police. They spot me every time. I reckon they park down the road and wait for me. Then they drive up to me. 'Hello Rile,' they say. 'Hop in.' And I do. I can't beat the buggers!"

Riley was on first-name terms with most of the local officers because he was such a regular passenger in their patrol cars. But it rarely occurred to him to take a less obvious route than the main road. Instead, he strode out in his signature 'Gonzo' walk along the most obvious route. His 'Gonzo' walk, adapted from a *Sesame Street* character, was his mannerism of walking stiffly and fast, arms rigid at his side, with his upper body extended forward, and his head and nose stuck out as far as possible.

But sometimes, his forays onto main roads had more serious intent than a simple bid for freedom. He walked against the traffic on the South-East Freeway in the hope that a car would hit him, and sometimes he stood at the side of a busy road with the intention of throwing himself in front of a truck. Of course we pleaded with him not to do this for his own preservation, but we also tried to impress on him the devastation his actions would cause an innocent motorist.

Sometimes his escapes were almost slapstick. Riley was in awe of the woman in charge of the psychiatric unit. "I was running away, Mum, high-tailing it down the hill and she chased me. She still had her high heels on and she had to take tibby steps because her skirt was so tight."

"Seeing as you are still here, Ril, I take it she caught you," I remarked.

"Yeah. She's amazing. How fast do you reckon she could run if she had the proper gear on?"

"Faster than you, son. Faster than you!"

Sometimes when he absconded though, he was not apprehended before he had visited the nearby railway station where his intention was to end his life under a train. On one occasion he was laying across the lines, waiting for a train to come along. But before this happened, the driver of a train coming from the opposite direction on parallel lines, saw him, stopped his train, and vehemently abused Riley.

"You should have heard his language, Mum. I'm not copping that! I'm going to report him for verbal abuse. He can't speak to the general public like that and I'm a general public! Who the hell does he think he is?" Cause and effect had no correlation in Riley's illogical thought processes.

Until becoming Dr Cooper's patient, Riley had never been prescribed medication. With the benefit of hindsight, however, it is difficult to say which was worse: Riley's behaviour without medication, or the devastating and destructive effects of the medication prescribed for him over the last four years of his life.

In his pre-medication days, Riley *was* plagued by delusions, ran away, regularly self-harmed, and attempted suicide frequently, but he was articulate, his handwriting was neat and legible, and his eyes were bright and focused. His spiral into absolute hell coincided with the commencement of prescription drugs. Everything that had been distressing in the past now became even worse. His speech became slurred and monosyllabic, his handwriting regressed to that of a young child learning to form big, shaky letters, his eyes were glazed and unfocused, we often had to feed him, he wet himself because he was so drugged, and he walked in a stiff, stilted gait. His stomach was distended, and he dribbled. His hands shook, his body trembled, and his skin sometimes came out in an itchy rash.

When his delusional state was at its worst, Riley was placed in solitary confinement, or 'conciliatory refinement' in Riley's idiom. It is a bare concrete, bunker-like room with an uncovered mattress on the floor, a fixed glass pane looking out to the garden, and a narrow slit of glass in the internal door through which nursing staff could look to check on him. The bathroom was behind a locked door and there was a red panic button on the wall. If Riley needed to use the toilet, he had to ring the panic button, but often the nurses were too busy to come to him in time. "I wet myself again today, Mum," he wept, ashamed and humiliated.

"It's the drugs, son. It's not you. You can't help it. It's okay."

One time when I visited him in solitary confinement, the staff could not find the key to let me into his room. I stood waiting while staff patted uniform pockets, looked under papers on the bench, and rummaged through drawers. How would he have fared if there had been a fire? I have a painful memory of Riley's face peering out at me through the glass slit, unable to understand why I was not coming in to him. Through the glass window that separated me from my son, I watched him mouthing, "Mum? Mum?"

We often had to feed Riley when he was heavily medicated because he couldn't do it himself. He at least had the shakes and spilt his food everywhere, or he was so drugged he couldn't find his mouth with the spoon – he was rarely given a knife and fork for safety reasons. And sometimes he was unaware that food had been placed in front of him. He slumped back against his pillows while his food went cold, dribble running down his chin.

At one stage, he developed a toxic reaction to his medication that made him itchy, twitchy, and blotchy. He was in a terrible condition. The only treatment was to keep up his fluid intake to flush the toxins from his body and this took a week to be effective. He lay prone on his bed, frantic with discomfort, while Kevin spent most of the week with him, trying to help with his care and ease his symptoms by constantly sponging him with cool cloths and massaging his legs and arms. I went up each evening after work and gave him head massages. In happier times when we were relaxing, he would sidle up to me and say, "Any chance of a head massage, Mum?" He almost purred like a kitten when I obliged.

Under the influence of his medication, he would curl up like a foetus and sleep a drugged sleep for excessive hours. He would wake up, take more prescribed tablets and go back to sleep. When he was on a home visit, I would stand by his bed, just as I had when he was an infant, and gaze at him, but now it was with despair and sorrow. 'How has my son come to this?' I asked myself. He was a physical wreck. His mental state continued to deteriorate and his suicide attempts became even more bizarre.

Riley climbed the Story Bridge three times with the intention of jumping to his death. I asked him once what stopped him from jumping.

"It was low tide," he replied. "There was mud below. I didn't want to get dirty." At the time of his death, he was on a charge for causing a public nuisance after another bridge climb and the inevitable traffic disruption this caused, because police had to close the bridge while a negotiator persuaded him to come down.

In the last year of Riley's life, he swallowed safety razor blades on three separate occasions. The first was surgically removed, and the other two were being monitored by x-rays. One was present in his body when he died.

Still searching for a positive replacement activity that would benefit Riley, Dr Cooper investigated the possibility of placing him in a supportive rural community where he might develop an interest in country life. I wondered if that onion furrow would ever become a reality! However, none of these communities were prepared to take on someone with the difficulties that Riley had. As well, the supervision of his potent medication was always a problem when Riley was away from the hospital environment. But regardless of whatever innovative ideas were tried, they were of no consequence because Riley's interest in new ventures consistently waned after about two weeks. And if he couldn't derail positive treatment strategies with disinterest, Riley had an uncanny ability to sabotage efforts that were made to rehabilitate him.

Another one of Dr Cooper's positive tactics was to encourage Riley to try 'transitional accommodation'. This was meant to give him the opportunity to live away from Keswick in a supported hostel that worked closely with Riley's medical team. His intermittent stays at this wonderful hostel under the care of Hilary, the landlady, were determined by his mental state: when he was fairly rational, he lived at Hilary's and when he was in a bad mental state, he returned to the hospital. And sometimes he came home for short periods.

Hilary called the male residents 'her boys'. She was a petite Irish woman with long grey hair that was always bunched up in an untidy bun. Wispy strands escaped and fell around her face. I admired Hilary's fortitude in dealing with 'her boys' on her own, as her husband was a merchant seaman and rarely at home to provide assistance or support.

Riley lived at Hilary's for longer than he lived in any other accommodation, but eventually she had to ask him not to return because he stole a radio from one of the neighbouring homes. As the proprietor of a home for mentally ill men, Hilary was mindful of maintaining good neighbourhood relationships so that the hostel would continue to be tolerated in the area.

I remember a senior nurse at Keswick throwing her arms in the air when she heard what Riley had done. "Sabotage," she said. "Every time we look like making some progress, he sabotages it. He won't let himself, or us, succeed." I knew exactly how she felt.

Although we had spent many years locking Riley *inside* our home to prevent him from absconding, in the last few years of his life, we were instructed on three occasions to lock him *out*. As his mind deteriorated even more, the staff at Keswick phoned to warn us that Riley had absconded, having declared first that he was going to kill his family. They had a legal obligation and duty of care to warn us, and instructed us to lock all doors, not to venture outside, and not to open the door to Riley if he arrived at home. And of course, we were told to phone the police if Riley arrived at home, or if we knew where he was. The police were informed that he was at large, and we were only to unlock ourselves after he had been detained. Quite apart from the hospital's warnings, the police informed us twice that Riley had made similar threats against us.

We never acted on these warnings as instructed, and went about our lives as normal. Perhaps we were nonchalant about the warnings because we had never been put to the test of Riley confronting us in any threatening way. Verbal abuse, yes. But physically, he was kind and gentle to everyone except himself. His fantasies were frightening, but Riley was not. I was frightened *for* Riley, not *of* Riley.

During these years, Riley's medication was always being altered and adjusted, but it was never right. Despite the doctor's perseverance and dedication in finding the elusive combination, we never had one scintilla of hope throughout this time whereby we thought his medication was having a beneficial effect. Consequently, in the final two years of Riley's life, I asked for him to be taken off all medication. "Just stop giving him tablets. Don't give him any more," I pleaded, begged.

"It doesn't work like that. His medication can't be stopped just like that. We've got to work on getting the right combination and balance," Once again I was told to be patient.

It was becoming increasingly obvious that his medication was not providing any relief from his mental illness. But by this time, Riley was heavily dependent on medication, and we were on a merry-go-round of delusional episodes and potent prescription drugs. Tragically, that merry-go-round turned into an out-of-control roller coaster. We were all going down hill at break-neck speed.

However, it is impossible to know how Riley's mental state might have progressed without medication. Perhaps his condition would have been even worse. Who can say? We will never know. One thing we are certain of, though, is that if Riley had not been a regulated patient under the care of Dr Cooper, he would have ended up in jail. His options were clear: the medical system or the criminal justice system, because our social and political structure does not provide for any other alternatives.

My pleading to have Riley taken off medication coincided with Riley being referred to a neurologist to have the functioning of his brain examined. Riley was so keen to have this procedure done, he insisted that we arrive early for the appointment – we had to settle in – and we passed the time until his appointment sitting on a park bench opposite the doctor's surgery. Riley had no doubt that at last this brain scan would reveal the underlying causes of his dysfunction.

Exuding optimism, he told me, "This is it, Mum! I can feel it in my bones! At last we are going to find out why I'm like this, why I've got problems! When they know what's wrong with my brain, they'll give me treatment and I'll be normal! Normal, just like other people, Mum! That's all I've ever wanted. My life will be different." His introspection and self-awareness broke my heart.

We crossed to the surgery, and as we sat in the waiting room Riley was restless with excitement, smiling a happy grin that I hadn't seen for a long time. Faced with such optimism, I didn't have the courage to dampen his spirits by suggesting caution about his expectations. Happiness and hope were such rare emotions for Riley; I couldn't bring myself to take these feelings away from him. And even I had a glimmer of anticipation that he might be right. Perhaps, I thought, just maybe, this scan will give us the answers that we've been searching for. Don't take away his hope unless it is absolutely necessary.

When the scan was completed, we went off in high spirits to have lunch before returning to the surgery in the afternoon for the results. But no neurological irregularities were detected and Riley crumpled at the news as we left the doctor's office. His shoulders sagged, his face was wooden, and his step was slow. His eyes had that glazed look of despair that I knew so well. He kept shaking his head in disbelief. "I feel let down, Mum. So let down." He was choking with emotion, his voice nothing more than a croaking whisper. Like us, he was desperate for a tangible explanation for his disordered conduct.

Although Riley lived for another two years, I believe that this news confirmed his opinion that his life was not worth living. "I'm not going to grow old, Mum. I'll never be thirty," he assured me.

Chapter 12

In the beginning, Riley's self-harm and suicide attempts distressed me to the point of hysteria, but, as the years passed, these repetitive episodes became almost normalised into our lives. It wasn't that we were blasé, but this is what we had to deal with on a daily basis for more than a decade. And we could do nothing to stop it despite our most concerted efforts.

I went through several phases of trying to dissuade Riley from his damaging behaviour. My initial bouts of hysteria always included telling him how much we loved him and how empty our lives would be without him. Then I tried persuasion, resorting to blackmail. "How will Grandma cope if you die? I'll tell you how. She'll die of a broken heart. Is that what you want? She adores you and she'll never understand." I even vented my anger and rage on him that he could inflict this life sentence on those of us who loved him and that we would be left to cope with the guilt and grief of his death. "Do you think your death will solve the problem? Well, it bloody well won't for your father and me and Coby. How do you think we'll cope? Have you given that any thought? I bet you haven't. Don't be so bloody self centred and selfish. There are others in this world apart from you." But, obviously, none of my ploys were heeded.

Information on ways to self-harm and methods of completing suicide is readily exchanged amongst psychiatric patients. Such behaviour is almost mandatory etiquette in a mental health culture. If a patient doesn't know how to do these damaging acts before entering hospital, they do once they are within the psychiatric system. Riley explained to me how to "correctly" complete a hanging, and how to effectively slash wrists.

"You don't do it like they show in the movies, Mum. That's rubbish." He was scornful. "You do it this way," he said, demonstrating with a trailing finger how to make the cut on his wrist.

I asked Riley many times how he endured the pain of such terrible mutilations. His replies were always the same. "I don't feel pain when I cut myself or whatever, only a terrific sense of relief. I feel calm. When I see blood flowing from my flesh, I know I exist. There is blood, so there must be life." He told me this in tones that might be expected if the soothing benefits of meditation was being discussed.

He added, "What you might feel as pain, is for me a wonderful feeling of pleasant release, like a boil bursting and all that pressure gushing out."

His psychiatrist explained to us that what dissipated for Riley was anger, frustration, and despair. He felt calm after these self-mutilations because he exorcised so much pent-up emotion. It is common for people who self-harm to become addicted to the exhilaration of the harm/relief cycle.

Riley concluded his explanation with a grumble about the medical people who treated his wounds. "It really hurts when the doctors start stitching me up or fixing my burns. That's when the pain begins. I wish they'd just leave me alone. They're interfering in my personal life. I don't want them poking their bibs in." He saw this medical treatment as external interference in his innermost torment, a torment that was private and personal, to be dealt with in his way of choosing. He would, as always, decide his own decides.

The daily routine in any of the hospitals where Riley spent time lacked stimulation and the boredom which permeated his every day provided him with ample opportunity to indulge in morose thoughts and self-harm.

While he was in Keswick, I regularly took Riley grocery shopping. The plan was simply to get him out of the hospital environment and to make him think that he had a purpose in helping me with a chore.

He often teased me by lingering in the dog food aisle: "I think she likes this one," he'd say as he picked out a particular brand of dog food.

"But you haven't got a dog, Ril." My dialogue in this little scene was well rehearsed.

"I know that! It's for my new girlfriend, Mum. Just thought I'd get her a bit of a snack." Political correctness was still a few years off.

"I hope she's nice, Riley, like that one that I took a shine to, you know, what's her name? The one whose tattoos were spelt correctly. I thought that was a big plus in her favour," I'd add to our gauche fun. We'd continue down the aisles, elbowing each other in a faux jostle.

But sometimes, for no apparent reason, his mood could change suddenly from amiable to abusive. He would come to a halt, glare at me through glazed eyes and snarl, "Stuff you." Then he would shove the trolley into the stacked shelves and storm off. I would abandon the trolley, step over cans and packets, and chase him through the centre. When I caught up with him, I'd have to physically grapple him, manhandle him into the car, and return him to the nearby hospital.

On some shopping trips, Riley invited his mate Jack along. Jack was also a patient at Keswick, and I found myself in the company of two young men whose potential for dysfunctional behaviour was unpredictable. Jack was a big blond, surfie type who was frank about his excessive marijuana use escalating into psychosis. He was a well-mannered, reticent lad, and he liked a good giggle.

My strategy on these shopping trips was to involve the two of them in the decision-making process of what I should purchase. "What do you think, boys? Green or yellow?" I held up T-shirts.

"Geez, Mrs Brasch, I reckon they'd both be good," Jack offered.

"Thanks, Jack. You're no help," I chided.

He giggled.

Riley seemed to relish my involvement with his mate and never behaved badly when we had Jack with us. Perhaps I should have kept Jack with us twenty-four hours a day! Nonetheless, as the three of us sat having a snack after the shopping was done, I felt that the circumstances were surreal. I sat back and looked at Riley and Jack, and thought how lovely this would be under normal circumstances. To a passer-by we were an ordinary threesome: a mother sharing a pleasant outing with her son and his mate. But the reality took me out of my reverie. The heartbreaking effects of mental illness are a nightmare and the nightmare had become my daily routine. I remember sitting there with them and thinking, 'Well, here I am. This is how it is. This is my life. I hope we all get home in one piece.'

Another patient who Riley took a shine to was Brad. Big Brad. "Bradley needs somewhere to live, Mum, when he's discharged next week. He can stay at our place, can't he? I've told him he's welcome. That's right, isn't it, Brad? You'll be right, mate. Mum and Dad will take care of you." Riley, ever the kind friend.

"Well, what say I have a chat to Bradley's doctor and see what he advises," I replied. "I've noticed Brad's mum visiting sometimes. I'm sure she'll want a say about where Bradley lives, too. We'll all make whatever decision is best for Bradley."

But, by the time it came for Bradley to be released, both he and Riley had forgotten the accommodation promise. I was proud of Riley's compassion for his fellow inmate, but did not see myself as the benevolent keeper of a halfway house. We couldn't manage our own son, so how would we cope with others?

In yet another feeble attempt to engage Riley in some sort of activity on my daily visits, I tried to interest him in doing 'Find the Word' puzzles. At first, I was successful and we worked on these for hours, but there are only so many words that can be found before the challenge fizzles out. One day I arrived at the hospital with a new 'Find the Word' book under my arm and Riley erupted. "Take your bloody Word book and bugger off. I'm sick of finding words. I never want to find another bloody word as long as I live." A simple 'No, thanks' or 'Not today, Mum,' would have done, I thought, as I took the Word book and myself home.

I could cope with this sort of rejection and could even have a chuckle at my own boringness, but there were other occasions when his rejection left me numb.

"Piss off! JUST! PISS! OFF!" His raised voice was muffled by the loud hum of the interval audience at the Lyric Theatre. Tinkling laughter. Clinking glasses. Sparkling city lights illuminated the night sky through the glass windows. Huddled in a corner. Arms wrapped tightly round his upper body. Back half-turned to me. Turned against the tittering theatre patrons. Turned against the world. His eyes were glazed with rage. His face was florid. He spat invective over his left shoulder at me.

"Bugger off. Why don't you just bugger off? Bugger out of my face, out of my sight, out of my life. Do me a favour. Just bugger off!"

"It's okay, Riley. It's okay. Let's just take our time. We don't have to go back in. We'll go home."

"Look at him! Look at him! And look at him!" He flung his arm in the direction of three young men with their female partners. "Look at me!" In a singsong voice, "I'm with my mummy. I'm with my mummy. The veggie's with his mummy."

"We'll go, Rile. When you're ready. We'll go home. To the hospital."

"Get stuffed!"

I put my hand out to him, hoping to make physical contact, hoping to turn him towards the exit. Towards the car. Towards the hospital. Towards shelter. He recoiled as if my fingers were stabbing daggers. He glared hatefully at me.

"You don't have to walk with me, son. Let's just try for the car. I can't leave you here. When you are safe, I'll go. I'll bugger off. But I have to get you home. The car, son. Can we try for the car? Please?"

The drive to hospital was silent, except for the breath that seethed through his clenched teeth. His back was turned to me. My lap was damp. Tears dripped from my chin.

I was at the front doors of Keswick. Big double glass doors. I pressed the night bell. A male nurse opened the door.

"Hello, Mrs Brasch. Riley. Have you had a good outing?"

"Not really." My voice quivered. The nurse made eye contact with me. No words were needed.

"We'll deal. 'Night, Mrs. Brasch. Take care." He led Riley inside and locked the glass doors.

I stood outside the glass doors and watched my son walk slowly down the long corridor. The nurse was not in my vision. Night lights gave the corridor an ethereal glow. My son's back was still to me. He was just a dark shape disappearing into the shadows. His head was down. His shoulders drooped. His step was jerky. He didn't look back. I watched until I could no longer see him.

Towards the end of Riley's life when he was most fragile, his mind was taking a terrible toll on him. "I keep having this same dream, Dad. I'm standing at the top of the stairs and my head falls off. It rolls down the stairs and blood is going everywhere. Up the walls, all over the stairs. Then my eyes fall out of my head. They roll down the stairs, too. But I'm still watching all this happening even though my head and eyes are at the bottom of the stairs."

Kevin and Riley were sitting amongst a crowd of people at a busy shopping centre. Kevin was familiar with this sort of revelation and sat quietly, listening. It was nothing new. But on this occasion, he became aware of the crowd thinning out around them. In a short time, Kevin and Riley were left alone like isolated islands. Had the uninitiated overheard Riley, and moved off, or was Kevin imagining things? But we knew that others, too, were unexpectedly shaken by Riley's deteriorating mind.

Narelle, my youngest sister, always supported Riley and included him in as much of her family life as possible. She, too, told him that she couldn't manage her weekly shopping without his help; she took him to her young son Ben's sporting fixtures; and Riley was always a guest at family barbeques. Riley loved Narelle and her husband Ross and enjoyed being with them. Their home was full of laughter. He was always well behaved on these outings and visits until one day when he was in the car with Narelle and Ben. Suddenly, Riley went into twitching, jerking spasms and started talking to 'Helen', the voice in his head. Narelle and Ben were frightened and after this experience, Narelle was dubious about taking Riley for further outings. Understandably, she felt that she couldn't risk exposing Ben to another episode of what they had both witnessed. Her account of Riley talking to Helen was familiar to me. I, too, had encountered Helen.

I had called at the hospital to collect Riley for an outing. I knew instantly that the evening would not go well because he was in a mood. He was agitated and withdrawn. Still, this was not uncommon. As we drove away from the hospital, I kept up a constant flow of prattle, thinking to diffuse the situation, but Riley seemed to be unaware of his surroundings and me. He was muttering to himself.

A few minutes into the drive, Riley suddenly appeared to convulse. He strained against his seatbelt. His torso and limbs were rigid, jerking and twitching. Within the confines of his passenger seat space, he was ducking and diving, weaving, jerking, contracting. His hands flickered to his face, away from his face, fingers stretched out stiff, rigid. Contorted.

I flung my left arm out to restrain him.

"What are you doing? Riley? What's happening? Stop it!" He seemed to be speaking to someone.

"Helen…coming...yes...there…"

It made no sense to me. I pulled the car off the road, released my seatbelt, twisted in my seat and grabbed his shoulders with both my hands. My impulse was to shake him back to reality. But he was still unaware of me and, in the confined space of the car, my physical efforts to restrain him were ineffectual. By now I was astride the hand brake, trying to get closer to him. The jerking rigidity continued. His eyes were rolled up. His body darted up and down. Jerky movements. Rapid movements.

"Yes, Helen, I hear you. Now. When? Yes. I hear. What? Blood. Helen. Yes, blood. Where? I'm coming. Now. Good. Bring you blood? Yes, I hear. Where you are? There? Come to you Helen. I'll come! Coming! Want to be with you. There." His chant went on and on, incoherent, babbled. I knew I was screaming, yelling, shaking Riley, afraid, confused. I didn't know what to do. Help was not at hand and I couldn't drive the car in these circumstances.

Suddenly, Riley sighed and sank back in his seat, exhausted, as if he had just finished a gruelling, physical task.

Tentatively, I spoke. "Riley? Riley? Son?" His tired eyes looked at me and he started to weep. As best I could I gathered him in my arms, cradled his head on my shoulder, and gently rocked him back and forth. We both cried softly.

"Was it Helen, Mum?"

"I think it might have been, son. You were saying 'Helen'. But it's over now. Take it easy."

"It was Helen, Mum. Helen."

He scrunched even more tightly against me. I wrapped him closer to me and made the soft noises mothers have made to calm their babies through eternity.

Later, when Riley seemed calmer, he explained: "Helen was someone I knew years ago. But she died. Now she's the voice that comes in my head. She's very strong, powerful. I must do what she says. I try not to Mum. Believe me. But I know before, when she's coming. I get a sensation." This explained the mood I detected at the start of my visit. He continued, "And I get frightened. I'm so scared. I try not to listen to her, Mum. But she's stronger than me. And she wants me to come to her."

"Come where, Ril?"

"There. There, Mum."

"What do you mean, There? Where's There? Where…is… There? I don't understand. You have to help me! Please!"

"I don't understand either, Mum. All I know is that Helen comes, a voice in my head, and she wants me with her. There. She says it's peaceful, beautiful. There."

"Riley, she's just a…a voice!…Nothing! Only your imagination. In your head! She's not real! There is not real! We're real. Here is real, Riley. Here! You and me!"

"No, Mum. Helen tells me There is better than Here."

"I have to get you back to the hospital, Riley." I was frightened. I did a u-turn and made a familiar, sorrowful trek back to where we had come from.

Chapter 13

Because Riley came under the control of the *Mental Health Act* as a regulated patient, it meant that even though we were his parents, we had to comply with the law when we wanted to interact with Riley. He could only be released into our care under certain conditions. Whenever we wanted to take him for an outing, or bring him home for a stay, we had to sign a legal form acknowledging our understanding of Riley's condition and accepting responsibility for him while he was in our care. But sometimes our responsibility was reduced to farce.

"I've got some business to do in the Valley, Ril, and then we'll have coffee and cake. Okay, son?" Kevin had signed the form to take Riley out for the day.

"Yup, I'm with you, Dad."

Later, when they were having coffee, Riley said that he needed to go to the toilet. Kevin let him go by himself, not thinking for a moment that this might present a problem. Some time passed and Riley didn't return. Kevin was suddenly startled, realising that he should not have allowed Riley to go off on his own. He rushed into the toilets to look for Riley.

"Are you there, Riley? Where are you, son? Riley! Riley, answer me!" He was nowhere to be seen, and did not respond to his name being shouted out, so Kevin got down on his hands and knees to look up into the closed cubicles in case Riley had self-harmed and was unconscious. A man came into the toilets, saw Kevin on the floor and froze, staring, his mouth gaping in shock. He turned and hastily retreated from the toilet block. Kevin too was gaping, offering unheard words of defence to the man's disappearing back. "But, my son…I can't find my son…" In the next instant, Kevin realised that this innocent but seemingly sordid scene could escalate into a bigger problem. He ran from the toilets in anticipation of the police being summoned and found Riley waiting patiently at their coffee table.

"Where've you been?" Kevin puffed while looking furtively for approaching constabulary. "I've been looking for you in the toilets and you weren't there. Where were you?"

"In there, Dad," Riley indicated the adjacent disabled toilet. "I *am* disabled, you know."

One of the decisions Riley made as a legal adult was to give his signed consent to have electric shock therapy (ECT). ECT involves the consenting patient being placed under a general anaesthetic, injected with a muscle paralysing agent and then having an electric current passed through their brain via electrodes fixed to the scalp. Kevin and I were distraught and made our objections known to the hospital staff, but we were powerless to stop the treatment.

A decade after Riley received his series of ECT, Institute of Australasian Psychiatrists Fellow Dr William Wilkie voiced his concerns that in Queensland's private psychiatric hospitals, "patients were twice as likely to receive ECT than patients in most other states." He added that some psychiatrists earned themselves the nickname 'Dr Zap', and while ECT was a legitimate treatment, "poor training and practising standards in Queensland meant the therapy was being abused."

Offering an alternative opinion to Dr Wilkie's criticisms, Associate Professor Gerard Byrne, Royal Australian and New Zealand College of Psychiatrists Queensland chairman, argued that "…the only people who want to have [ECT] are those that are seriously ill."

But how can someone who is "seriously ill" make an objective judgement that they want ECT? And how could someone as impaired and seriously ill as Riley understand what he was giving his consent to? It was only after his first ECT treatment that he realised what was involved. Although we begged him to revoke his permission for ECT, he refused. This was yet another way of harming himself. His only concession to the horror of ECT was to ask his father to be present on each of his treatment days, which Kevin tried to do. Mostly though, the nursing staff did not allow Kevin near Riley when he was being prepped for treatment, but Kevin turned up anyhow.

Kevin anticipated each treatment day with dread and returned home distressed. "I don't know what to do, Til. It's awful. If the staff let me, I sit with him before he has the ECT, and I stay with him when they take him back to his bed. I just hold him. It's horrible. It breaks my heart."

Although Riley was borderline mentally retarded, of low intellect, delusional, and heavily medicated, once he turned eighteen, the law allowed him to make the decision to have ECT. And his legal right to do so was sustained by his medical team.

Continuing to exercise his rights, Riley regularly drew up contracts that had legal standing, preventing his father and me from having contact with him. These documents were counter-signed by members of his medical team: his psychiatrist, and his case manager. Then Kevin and I were required to sign also as acknowledgement of the contract. In part, a formal Agreement on Riley's Living Arrangement composed by his case manager read:

> ***Contact with Parents***
>
> *With immediate effect of the signing of this agreement, contact with parents will be through telephone only for the following four weeks. Demands and needs felt by either parties to get together will have to wait until the month is over and Riley's emotional status consequent to this new arrangement is evaluated with him. The same arrangement or variations of it may be renewed at the end of the one-month period.*

Attached to this document was a personal note from Riley:

> *Dear Mum and Dad,*
>
> *I am writing you this letter to clarify a few points.*
>
> *The visitation rights are not for a nother 3 months*
>
> *No telephone contact on your part*
>
> *$15.00 into my account + the rest into my bank account*
>
> *As the contract stands with Ann Porter the 3 month period stands as from the date signed by 1 myself Ann Porter Dr Cooper and Mises T Brasch.*
>
> *If Dad wants to take any Legal action I am more than willing to come to the party.*
>
> *PS Photo Copy a copy for Dad.*

How meaningful was it for the law to allow Riley to make these decisions? Because of statutes that protected Riley's position as a legal adult, choices about his life defaulted to various busy medical professionals to the exclusion of his concerned and committed family. In effect, our son was ours biologically, but not legally. There was something in this that reminded me of the frail nursery once again.

In the years after Riley died, Queensland implemented legal reforms to address this anomaly by enacting the *Guardianship and Administration Act 2000* for 'assisted and substituted decision making' in the case of adults with impaired decision-making capacity. If this law had been available when Riley was alive, Kevin, Coby, and I could have made a simple application to the Guardianship and Administration Tribunal to be allowed to at least assist Riley with personal and financial decisions, if not make those decisions on his behalf.

But for the duration of Riley's illness, we were constrained by complex and restrictive laws, which protected his legal status in spite of his mental incapacity.

However, despite significant legal barriers which would have involved the Supreme Court, in the last months of Riley's life, processes were being put in place to legalise his guardianship through a family *Committeé* as a way of preventing Riley from making inappropriate medical decisions and legalising my control of his finances. This *Committeé* would also allow designated family members the right to be informed not only about Riley's medical condition and treatment, but also about his admissions and discharges from hospitals. But he died before the process was completed.

We had avoided pursuing legal guardianship at an earlier period in Riley's life because we felt that removing his legal status would leave him with nothing — he would be a non-person — and we knew that he felt strongly that he should be allowed to decide his own decides.

But with the passing of time and the unfolding of events, we came to the conclusion that we had no other choice but to take this step. As always, our motivation was to protect Riley, even from himself. Giving legal rights to someone as mentally ill as Riley is tantamount to giving autonomy to a toddler.

Chapter 14

While Riley was in Keswick, we tried to have our own versions of positive replacement therapy by constantly varying his life as a way of stimulating interest in his otherwise negative routine. We wanted him to have events and outings to look forward to, and plans to make. If a concert, festival, or an adventure came to our notice that might interest Riley, we went along, like the time Riley and I took a steam train day trip through the Brisbane Valley. A sunny spring day sheltered beneath a parasol of clear blue skies. The smell of burning coal, the hiss and puff of steam, and the hypnotic rhythm of wheels on tracks transported us back to another time. As we chuffed along, I told Riley stories about travelling on steam trains when I was a child.

At one stage early in the trip, the train had to climb a steep ascent at a speed slower than walking pace. Along with other passengers, Riley and I got out and walked through the bush alongside the snail-paced train. Our noses filled with bush smells from leaves crushed beneath our feet. Then, halfway through the journey, we alighted at a country town and watched the engine take on water at an ancient tank-stand. At the driver's invitation, Riley climbed into the engine's cabin and pulled the lever to send out a long, wailing whistle, which reverberated through the rural serenity.

At the furthermost point of our journey, we stopped in a little country town for a pub lunch.

"Any chance of a beer, Mum?" he asked as I ordered our steak sandwiches. The day had been so enjoyable and agreeing to his request seemed like a small gesture that I knew would add to his pleasure. How could I refuse? The rule about never mixing alcohol and medication slipped my relaxed mind.

After lunch, we strolled down the main street and inspected quaint little shops that were locked in a colonial time warp. Then we stretched out on the lawn under the shade of a tree that also shaded the obelisk honouring the district's fallen soldiers. This prompted a conversation between Riley and me about my late father, Riley's grandfather, a proud war veteran.

Then it was time for the homeward journey. On the way home, Riley curled up on the seat with his head on my lap and slept. He was contented, but I felt an underlying sense of melancholy about this special day. My heart yearned to hold on to the happiness we had shared, to never let it go, but experience told me that this was not possible: chaos would replace contentment when Riley gave in to the compulsion to punish himself for enjoying a pleasant outing. I knew that within a day or two, he would either disappear, refuse to have contact with us; mutilate himself; or attempt suicide. Happiness was always sabotaged.

Sometimes though, Riley tried to return the favour and entertain us. As a gift, Riley got his father to buy two tickets so that he could take me to see *Phantom of the Opera.* Around the same time, he also went to see a Michael Jackson concert with Coby.

"*Phantom* was much better than Michael Jackson, Mum. And at least you behaved yourself. You should have seen Coby at the Michael Jackson concert. She went ballistic, dancing and singing, jumping up and down on her seat. She was yelling and yahooing. Boy, it was embarrassing. I sat on my seat and hoped no one knew I was with her. She was very undignified, you know." I congratulated myself, pleased that I had done well in the dignity test.

As a young lad, Riley had been happiest and most carefree when he was on beach holidays at Tugun, a regular event in our family for thirteen years. Here, he seemed to revel in his freedom from schoolyard bullies, and the restrictions on his life did not intrude on his enjoyment of the beach and the surf where he frolicked like a young pup. We also formed close friendships with two other families who holidayed each year during the same three weeks as we did. The children of the three families became mates and shared happy times together.

As an adult, when life overwhelmed him, as it regularly did, Riley would take himself off to Tugun, his haven in times of trouble. Personal comfort was never of any consequence to him, and he happily slept rough in the local bus shelter or on a bench in a beachside park until he felt ready to come home, or until we found him.

To compensate for his long stay in Keswick, we made sure that we took him away on holidays as often as possible. One Christmas, at his request, we rented a beachfront unit for three weeks at his beloved Tugun. But at the last moment Riley refused to come with us. He sent us this letter:

> *Dear Mum & Dad,*
>
> *I am wrighting you this letter to you so we can come to some agreement or understanding. (1) I am spending Christmas in hospital, and their is no nagotiating on that subject, so just accsept it and forget it. The same goes for the Beach. I know the majority of things I do are related to self harm but they are ment to heart me and not you. The son you have is in those photographs, not the one in hospital.*

Despite our efforts to persuade him to come with us, and assurances from the staff at Keswick that it would be a good break for him, he spent Christmas in hospital. We had grown accustomed to his determination not to allow himself any sort of pleasure or enjoyment. Not coming to the beach or enjoying Christmas with us was another form of compulsive self-harm: emotional self-harm.

On yet another beach holiday organised for Riley, he came with us for a few days and then insisted on being taken back to hospital. He had reached the stage of panicking when he was away from the hospital environment. It was apparent that he was institutionalised and only felt safe within the confines of a hospital, even though he hated such places.

During these few days at the beach, we took him for just one walk in the late afternoon — that twilight period when day is all but over and night has not yet arrived. His doctor had warned us not to expose him to sunlight because his medication made his skin hypersensitive. Within a short time he complained, "Mum, my legs are itchy."

I had a quick look but saw nothing of concern. Perhaps there were sea lice in the water, I thought. He was wading at the edge of the waves. Shortly his complaint was more insistent.

"My whole body is itchy and tingly. I feel like I'm going to explode." He was frantically scratching and twitching.

I detected a red rash and it was obvious that Riley was more than uncomfortable. We found a tree to shelter under, and while Riley and I waited there, Kevin ran back to our accommodation to fetch the car. By the time he returned, Riley was a puffy red ball of itch and rash. He was in a state of collapse and had difficulty breathing. We phoned Keswick Hospital and from the symptoms we explained, they diagnosed hypersensitivity to the sun brought on, of course, by the effects of his medication. We should have been more careful. On the hospital's advice, we put him in a bathtub of water that we had chilled with ice until the rash subsided. He was exhausted and slept for hours. And even though we were at the beach, he could not swim, as his medication and the ocean were a dangerous combination.

It's hard to think of what pleasure there was in life for Riley during these years. A constant repetition of delusions, medication, and side effects to the medication dictated the limits of his life.

When Riley was on leave from the hospital, it was an impossible task for him to negotiate normal social exchanges with our well-meaning friends. Trying to make conversation with him, they usually asked him what he was presently doing or what had he been up to. These questions would seem to be reasonable, but what could he say? If he told the truth, he would have to say, "I'm on medication that would slow a bull-elephant down. I wet myself and dribble because of the medication. I can't put food in my mouth without spilling it because I've got the shakes." Or "I spent this week in isolation in a psychiatric hospital, on a bare mattress in a concrete room with only a slit of fixed glass to look out of." Perhaps he could tell them, "I had electric shock treatment again this week." Or maybe he could recount how inventive he had been with numerous ways to do himself harm, or attempt suicide. Instead, he recounted his fantasies, to meet what he saw as an appropriate social response.

"So, I haven't seen you in ages, Ril. What have you been up to?" A seemingly innocent question from a long-time family friend.

"Well, I've been doing a lot of track work for one of Brisbane's leading horse trainers lately. Had a few rides and a few wins. It's going okay. If he gets one of his horses into the Melbourne Cup, I'll mostly likely be the jockey. Yeah. Probably going to Melbourne for trials next week."

"Really? Let me know if you ride in the Cup and I'll put a bet on your horse."

How could he normalise this routine into friendships with well-intentioned people who didn't understand the day-to-day tragedy of someone with a mental illness? We had some overseas friends who wanted to visit him in hospital on one of their visits. "Please don't bring them to the hospital, Mum. I don't want them to see me as a veggie," he begged.

Apart from being imaginative, Riley's delusions could sometimes be somewhat melodramatic. In some of his fantasies, he saw himself in the role of a Hollywood Hero who holes up against the world. In one of his lucid periods, and while on leave from hospital, Riley hired a utility from the Gold Coast to help someone shift furniture, but when he realised that the time for returning it had passed, instead of doing something logical like return it and pay a late fee, he thought his only option was to make a run for it. In his mind, he was 'on the run from the cops.' He was certain that the police would be looking for the ute as a stolen vehicle and decided to head for the Glass House Mountains, north of Brisbane, barricade himself in a cave, and defend himself with a gun (which he didn't have) against the inevitable police attack. But he was picked up in the city after running a red light, and a vehicle check soon revealed the status of the utility. This resulted in one of his overnight stays in a watch-house cell and a later court appearance. We were not informed that he was in the watch-house. We found out a few days later when Riley told us how terrified he was that another man being held in the same cell might rape him.

The most ambitious idea that we had about positive therapy was to give Riley the experience of overseas travel, like other family members had enjoyed. But Dr Cooper didn't approve and cautioned us about the wisdom of travelling to Club Med in Noumea with Riley. However, once he realised that we were determined to make the trip, he did provide us with an official letter and medical documentation in case Riley had a delusional episode or fell foul of authorities with behaviour that broke local laws. It was difficult enough confronting the legal system on our home ground, but if this happened in a foreign country we could be in serious trouble. I also had a letter to authorise the vast amount of potent drugs that I took with me to cover all medical contingencies, and detailed instructions about what action to take if any one of myriad medical emergencies should happen.

Before we left, Dr Cooper's final caution to Riley was about the wisdom of having eight ear-studs along his ear. He said this would attract the attention of customs people and it would subject us to searches and 'agro'. But Riley refused to remove the studs.

We were tense as we went through customs on departure, but no one paid any attention to Riley's ear adornments. Thinking to circumvent possible trouble later in the trip, Kevin had a quiet word with one of the customs officials. He asked him to pull Riley aside and question him about his earrings. "Give him a bit of a shake up about the earrings. You know, let him know that they attract the wrong sort of attention."

A tap on the shoulder and a beckoning index finger indicated that Riley should step out of the line. "So, young man, what's with the earrings? How many have you got in there? Eight? Do I count eight?"

"Yes, I've got eight," Riley replied. "I just like them, that's why I wear them."

"Well, that's okay then. For a moment there I thought you were trying to smuggle earrings out of the country!" He threw his head back and laughed at his own joke. But the joke was on us.

We were spending ten days at Club Med. It was an easy, relaxed destination, which didn't put Riley under any pressure to meet daily itinerary schedules.

He and I had a lovely day visiting another island by catamaran for a barbeque lunch. The mostly Japanese female tourists on this trip tittered and giggled at Riley decked out in snorkel, goggles, and flippers while he was still dressed in day clothes, sitting at the back of the boat like a rear-end figure head. He didn't have his swimmers on because he couldn't go in the water. But they thought he was cute and funny and he played up to them.

Overall, the holiday was just a change of venue with the usual routines: Riley took medication and slept long hours while Kevin and I dispensed medication and watched over him. And Riley was so heavily medicated most of the time, he didn't have a clue where he was — he could have been on the moon or in Muckadilla.

But he did do some duty-free shopping on the way home, and bought a wristwatch, which managed to avoid the usual destiny of loss, swap, or trade-off. The watch was given back to us after his death, and it is a treasured possession for Kevin and me.

Chapter 15

After treating Riley for almost four years, Dr Cooper removed himself from Riley's medical team, deeming that a fresh perspective would be beneficial to Riley. He referred Riley to Dr Jensen. We were not consulted prior to this change in Riley's treatment, only informed after the event.

Kevin and I had just one consultation with Dr Jensen, who I found to be formal and unfriendly. He was rigid of stature and rigid in his manner with us. Two weeks after Riley became his patient, Dr Jensen phoned our home one evening. "I am no longer Riley's doctor," he announced. "No patient threatens my life and continues to be cared for by me." He didn't have the fortitude and patience of Dr Cooper.

Riley was abruptly cut adrift, removed from the security of a familiar doctor and taken out of Keswick Private Hospital, which had effectively been his home for almost four years. He was thrust back into the public health system feeling, like Kevin and me, frightened and unsure of the immediate future. In a little more than two months, Riley was dead.

Following his eviction, Riley was sent to a major public psychiatric unit for two days. He was then dispatched to an inner city hostel with the promise of support from a visiting case manager to help him cope. But this never happened even though the owner/manager of the hostel told us that he phoned the hospital several times, urging them to visit Riley because he was in a fragile mental state. The hostel was clean and efficiently administered and it seemed to me to be a good place, but after only a few weeks there, Riley left abruptly. Something happened which upset him, but he would not reveal what it was.

Two weeks and four days before Riley died, police removed him from bushland near our home because he had attempted to cut his throat. Again. Someone walking in the bush saw him covered in blood and alerted police. This was the second time police had intervened in an act of self-harm in four weeks. However, Riley was not kept at the public psychiatric unit where they took him, not even for observation. He was sent with great haste by the hospital social worker to Palmer Lodge hostel accommodation.

I found out about the incident in the bush and Riley's tenancy at Palmer Lodge from the manager of the hostel, who was keen to establish financial arrangements about Riley's board and lodging with me. Neither the police nor the hospital contacted me to tell me what had happened. I was angry and bewildered when I phoned the social worker at the hospital.

"Do you know how I found out what my son did this morning and where he is now? I found out from the manager of the hostel you've sent him to. Can you imagine what that feels like? It's hard enough to know Riley has tried to kill himself again, but to find out from a stranger who is only interested in how he is going to get his hands on Riley's dollars is wrong. Wrong, do you hear me? Do you care?"

"I'm sorry, Mrs Brasch, but you know all too well that that is the law. I don't make the laws and Riley didn't give us permission to notify you," she responded.

Most of the time when Riley was taken to public hospitals because he had harmed himself, his injuries were so severe and he was so heavily medicated, he would not have been capable of making a decision about who should or should not be informed. The law excluded us nonetheless. Good sense or compassionate consideration rarely prevailed.

"Well, why isn't he in hospital?" I continued. "Why hasn't he been detained? He's just tried to kill himself again. Again! How many times does he have to do this before you keep him in hospital instead of packing him off to a hostel? He needs treatment. He needs to be kept under observation. Why isn't the hospital caring for him?"

"Mrs Brasch, there is a bed shortage. We have no option but to prioritise."

Two weeks and four days later, my son died.

Several years later, Palmer Lodge was exposed by *Sixty Minutes* as a hostel of long-standing fraudulent management practices, poor hygiene, and substandard care policies.

Well-run, supported accommodation that provides a professional level of care for the mentally ill is a rare gem in our community and it is almost impossible to get a room in one of these better boarding houses. But sleazy accommodation, which is provided by morally deficient predators who see mentally ill people in terms of earning a quick and easy dollar, is readily available.

Riley stayed at Palmer Lodge for two weeks and four days before he died. Palmer Lodge filled us with despair. It was a dreadful place. We begged him to come home, but he was adamant that he wished to be independent. Something better would come up, he assured us. "This is just temporary," he promised. He spoke about going to Toowoomba or to the Salvation Army Hostel at Red Hill, but when he made this known to the manager of Palmer Lodge, he was told he could forget any idea of leaving. "There's only one way people leave here mate, and that's in a pine box," he told Riley. This threat came true. The manager controlled the residents with fear and intimidation.

I never met the manager, Mr Stewart, in person. He was always unavailable when I visited Palmer Lodge and asked to see him. I could only make contact with him by phone and he made it clear from the outset that he didn't want to deal with me. "What say I talk to hubby, love?" he asked in our initial phone conversation about Riley's board and lodging.

"I look after Riley's finances, Mr Stewart. If you want to be paid, you'll deal with me."

"Yeah? So what's wrong with hubby, then? Can't he get his hands on the purse strings or something?"

"Nothing is wrong with my husband. He looks after some aspects of Riley's life and I take care of Riley's finances. That's how it is."

"Is that so?" he sniggered.

Mr Stewart was not the owner, only the manager of Palmer Lodge. The conversation continued with an instruction for me to have Riley's Disability Support Pension signed over to him, "like the other residents do."

"That sounds highly irregular to me, Mr Stewart. I won't be doing that. As I have already told you, I look after Riley's affairs."

"Okay, if that's how it's going to be. These are my personal bank account details and I want you to deposit Riley's fortnightly payments into this account."

"Shouldn't the money be paid into a Palmer Lodge account, some sort of business account?" I asked.

I could hear his angry breathing through the phone. "Don't you bother yourself about that, lady. I run this business, not you."

Kevin described Mr Stewart as a big man who wore unbuttoned shirts that hung open over his rotund stomach. He had a gravelly voice and was always unshaven. A limp roll-your-own cigarette seemed to be permanently stuck to his bottom lip. He wore thongs on his feet even though it was almost winter.

On my first visit to Palmer Lodge, Riley showed me around. As I walked through the rabbit's warren of rooms on the lower floor, my nose stung with the smell of disinfectant. The rooms were airless and dim. The floors were painted concrete, scattered with sparse plastic furniture. Plastic ribbon strips hung at the doors to keep out insects. Outside was a dirt yard. Little tufts of grass struggled for survival.

Upstairs was a maze of bedrooms, but I had to concede that Riley's bed did look comfortable and warm. Riley shared the bedroom with a man who had just been released from prison. Riley introduced me to him and his leering look made my skin crawl. His mouth hung half open with wet, sloppy lips. I walked away in an effort to avoid him, but he skulked after me, still leering through half-closed eyes. I shivered. I never asked what he had been in prison for. I thought it best that I didn't know. After this first meeting, when I called to take Riley out, this man always followed and ogled me. To avoid this, I arranged for Riley to meet me on the footpath, but the man was always there, in the yard and on the footpath, just staring at me. On occasions when I had no option but to enter the premises, I was frightened. We would not allow Coby to go to Palmer Lodge because we felt it was not safe.

In the short time that Riley was at Palmer Lodge, Kevin and I took every opportunity to take him on outings or bring him home just to get him away from this awful place. The hostel wasn't far from the beach and Kevin and Riley sometimes just walked along the foreshores or up to the nearby shopping village for coffee. But Mr Stewart didn't approve of our presence and encouraged Riley to sever contact with us. "I'll take care of you, mate. I know the ropes. You don't want to hang around with your folks, do you?"

Mr Stewart continued with his efforts to alienate Riley from us and relationships soured even further when Kevin eventually challenged him. "We will see our son as often as we want to. We will handle his affairs. This is how it has always been done and will continue to be done in the future. Your expertise is not required, thank you."

On one occasion when I called for Riley, I had to collect his medication from the young girl who had been left in charge. She was on her own, just a young teenager, dressed in a short skirt and skimpy top. Riley watched as she placed his medication in my hand.

"They're not right, Mum – that's not what I take," he volunteered.

The girl got flustered.

"Here, let me do it," Riley said, and stepped in to sort out his tablets. The lass looked on as Riley read labels and counted tablets. The table was littered with unsecured bottles of medication.

"What nursing qualifications do you have?" I asked her.

"None," she said, without a trace of defence. "I just come in for a few hours sometimes to mind the place while Bill's not here. And to help get the tea ready."

I was shocked. If there were laws about this, they were ignored at Palmer Lodge.

On the day before Riley died, I paid his rent for the next two weeks into the manager's personal account. Following Riley's death, Coby made a request to the manager for the rent to be refunded, but the request was refused. Mr Stewart said that food had already been purchased in expectation of Riley being there for the following fortnight, and as his death had caused other residents great distress, he had called in a counsellor to assist them with their grief. He deemed that Riley's advance rental should pay for this. The money was of no consequence to us, but we were determined to expose how Mr Stewart was applying his defenceless tenants' dollars to his own account, even after death. To this end, we enlisted the support of the local parliamentary member, and only after months of distressing confrontation, did the manager begrudgingly consent to refund half the rental money, which we donated, to Rosie's Mission. However, we were deeply touched that the grief-stricken residents erected a white wooden cross in Gilmour Park where Riley died.

Riley's experience with the public mental health system was consistently one of superficial medical treatment, and of being discharged from hospital too quickly. And the hostels where hospital social workers place the mentally ill upon their discharge are mostly substandard places like Palmer Lodge that function to exploit the vulnerability of fragile people.

I asked the social worker who sent Riley to Palmer Lodge, "Have you inspected this hostel? Do you know what it is like? Do you know how it is run?"

"No," she replied. "We don't have the time to do inspections. But there are standards, and we do have to trust the people who provide accommodation. Sometimes we are desperate to find shelter for the people we are discharging and we have no options," she confessed.

In December 2003, *The Courier-Mail* reported on a run-down, filthy home for the mentally ill in South-East Queensland that was found to be "without toilets, bedding and hot water". This was despite the fact that, "Mental health workers visited the hostel weekly but nothing was done to improve conditions". In yet another respectable-looking home located in an affluent middle-class area on Bribie Island, "residents were beaten, tied to toilets, publicly humiliated and chemically restrained using unprescribed medication."

These practices strip people like Riley of dignity. They are made to feel worthless and that their future is hopeless. If the life they have lived to this moment is an omen of their future, they must ask, 'What's the point?'

Chapter 16

The prevalence of mental illness in modern societies is a silent statistic that is mostly under-estimated or ignored. In general, attitudes of the general population seem to reflect a desperate hope that, if they don't speak about mental illness, then it won't happen to them or their loved ones. But mental illness knows no boundaries of class, race, creed, gender, or age. And mental health is on the bottom rung of the health funding ladder.

Coby delivered a paper on the 'Human Rights of Mental Illness' in New York in 2003. Her research revealed these statistics: one in five Australians will have some form of mental illness at some stage in their life, while more than two million Australians will experience a mental illness each year. In Queensland, it is estimated that 2.9 per cent of the adult population suffers from a severe mental illness. This translates to 70,000 Queenslanders. Not included in these figures are homeless and itinerant people and some prison inmates who do not come to the attention of mental health authorities. The criminalisation of mental illness happens when mentally ill people are denied appropriate medical care and are more often than not turned away from hospitals to be swept up by the criminal justice system. Add to these figures the accumulative emotional and economic consequences that mental illness has on families, loved ones, friends, and employers and the insidious pervasiveness of mental illness becomes a fact which is in urgent need of attention from public and private sectors. But, because of the prejudice and stigma associated with mental illness, it is a tragedy that is unheard by those who have the power to make a difference to this vulnerable minority.

In September 1997, four months after Riley's death, Kevin and I attempted to present submissions about our concerns for the treatment of the mentally ill in Queensland to the State Minister for Health, but initially he would not grant us an appointment. It was only after the intervention of a senior reporter from Brisbane's *The*

Courier-Mail who always championed minority causes that we were given the opportunity to meet with the Minister. He accepted our submissions, spoke sympathetically with us, and gave an undertaking to look into the issues we raised. The outcome? Nothing.

In 2000, three years after Riley died, we were still campaigning for the rights of the mentally ill and wrote to the Premier of Queensland, Peter Beattie, and other State politicians, detailing our continuing concerns for the way this State fails to provide adequate health care and support facilities for its mentally ill population. In his reply to our correspondence, Mr Beattie admitted that his government had inherited a "legacy of neglect" and he acknowledged "that much more still needs to be done" in the mental health sector.

In early 2004, Brisbane's Wesley Hospital closed its psychiatric ward. Concerned people who protested about the closure asked, "Where do we go now?" In 1992, there were forty psychiatric beds per 100,000 Australians. By 2004, this ratio has been significantly depleted. Our personal experience is that when a hospital bed is not available for a psychiatric patient, that person is either sent home without adequate support, to an inappropriate hostel, or they are forced to live on the streets, and in some instances, these people die.

Responses received from other politicians we wrote to during our protest campaign in 2000 either repeated Mr Beattie's words, or we received a letter acknowledging receipt of our correspondence and nothing else happened.

More recently, on 19 January 2005, *The Courier-Mail* reported in an article, 'Hospital closes mental health beds', the reality of mental health services in Queensland:

"Queensland Health has indefinitely closed 15 per cent of mental health beds at Brisbane's Princess Alexandra Hospital because 100 per cent occupancy last year caused a $600,000 budget over-run."

This logic is difficult to follow, but even more bewildering are the financial facts. Mid 2004, Princess Alexandra Hospital opened its new $10.4 million mental health facility, but after nine months of full capacity, it closed 10 beds because of a $600,000 budget shortfall in a State where the Treasurer's State Budget 2004-05 forecasts a cash surplus of $1.059 billion, following a cash surplus forecast of $152 million for the previous period of 2003-04. Overflowing coffers. People in coffins.

While the Princess Alexandra management protested that, "it's good corporate governance to balance both the health service delivery and the allocation of dollars," concerned citizens, psychiatrists, and leaders of disability groups claimed that the closure of the psychiatric beds amounts to nothing more than a cost-cutting exercise which placed the lives of mental health consumers at risk. Queensland Alliance of Mental Illness and Psychiatric Disability Groups executive director said that, "Queensland had the lowest per capita expenditure for mental health of any state or territory [in Australia]." The director continued, "Mental health represents 30 per cent of all illnesses that occur, whereas less than 10 per cent of funding goes to mental health." Much more does need to be done.

Indeed, in March 2005, The Royal Australian and New Zealand College of Psychiatrists estimates that, "at a federal level alone, mental health is underfunded by as much as $2 billion."

According to Father Peter Nordern of Victoria's Catholic Social Service Secretariat, "more often than not politicians and the community at large pretend [the mentally ill] do not exist," and because "primitive fears about mental illness are still rife in society…its stigmatisation makes it hard to convince politicians that society's priorities [should] include the huge expenditure required to meet our goals". The goals referred to are those that give mental health consumers basic human rights in accordance with minimum standards as stipulated by the United Nations' *Principles for the Protection of Persons with Mental Illness*, adopted in 1991. In 1992, all Australian Health Ministers endorsed the *Principles* but Queensland failed to implement the standards for another decade, leaving its antiquated *Mental Health Act* (1974), which was based on the *English Lunacy Act*, unamended until February 2002.

Dr Grace Groom and Professor Ian Hickie, authors of *A Review of Mental Health Services in Australia – 2003: 'Out of Hospital, out of Mind!'* report that although combined Australian government expenditure for mental health has increased over the last decade to $778 million, this amount represents only half that of other first-world countries – seven per cent of overall health funding compared with 14 per cent. Consequently, the *Review* concluded that Australia still does not have a system of effective or accessible mental health care, and that "untreated mental illness is a leading contributor to Australia's suicide rate". However, the authors concede that the inadequate funding "does not represent a failure of policy but rather a failure of implementation through poor administration, lack of accountability, lack of ongoing government commitment to genuine reform and failure to support the degree of community development required to achieve high quality mental health care outside of institutional settings". Speaking to the *Review* in a parliamentary address on 12 November 2003, Clover Moore, Independent Member for the Federal electorate of Bligh, said: "Another issue is that many reports on mental health show that mental health funds are being allocated to cover for other health services, and that there is sleight-of-hand in reporting on mental health funds… No-one can assess these claims because there is a dearth of information about services and needs, and the extremely limited data published is years out of date".

These facts and figures come as no surprise to us. As a family, we were only too aware of the lack of funding, lack of beds, lack of resources, lack of community empathy, and lack of political morality that the mentally ill had to endure. For Riley and his family, there were never any perceptible benefits, support, or resources evident in his daily struggle that resulted from government funding.

This is how it was when we first engaged with the public mental health system in the early 1980s. This is how it is in 2005.

Chapter 17

Riley died during the cold, wet night of 16 May 1997, and I wasn't with him. He was two months away from his twenty-sixth birthday. After his countless suicide attempts and our many trips to hospitals and intensive care wards where Riley was mended after harming himself, I accepted the inevitability of his death, but I always thought that I would be with him at the end. I never contemplated that I would not hold him in my arms and whisper my good-bye.

My last physical contact with Riley was the day after Mother's Day, five days before he died. As a family, we had celebrated at lunch in the city and enjoyed a leisurely stroll through the Botanical Gardens on our way back to the car. It was a mild autumn day with blue cloudless skies. We farewelled Coby and then Kevin, Riley, and I drove to a nearby country town, and wandered around the craft shops. Riley was patient while I peeked into every corner and turned over each item. He engaged the storekeepers in conversation about their crafts, complimenting them on their skills, asking how long an item took to make, or how many could be made in a week. I recall him admiring a crinoline doll toilet roll cover. "It's lovely. Mum could do with one of these." I shot him an anxious glance.

Then we visited a Sunday market, and did some shopping at a plant nursery on the way home. He leapt to my assistance when I accidentally backed the car onto a fallen log, taking great pleasure in asserting his authority to help me out of a tight spot.

"Hard left, Mum. Don't rev it. Gentle. Gentle. No. You're spinning the tyres. Easy with the accelerator."

"Have I done any damage to the car, Ril?"

"Negative, Mother. Nnnnnegative!"

In his rational moments, Riley assumed a protective role with me and liked to think that I depended on him. In particular, I always got plenty of driving advice, and even now I use my indicators excessively in remembrance of his admonishment for the turns I made without indicating. "See that little lever there, Mum? Up for left, down for right. It's very nobble [Riley's word for novel]. Works every time and saves the bloke behind you guessing where you're going. But hey! Why let them know where you're going when, with no effort at all, you can confuse them? Is that the plan? Keep them guessing? 'Make my day. Guess where I'm going'?" He answered his own question.

And I don't cut corners. "That's your side of the road, Mum. What are you doing over here? Trying to get cosy with the oncoming traffic?"

"Don't get smart with me, Rile. I'm your mother, and I know about things," was my usual retort.

I last spoke with Riley on the phone Friday evening, 16 May, at 5.20pm. Specific details are important when memories are all you have left. Riley's voice was flat. He seemed detached and didn't have much conversation to offer. He sounded depressed, which was not unusual, but he had a cold with a bad cough, and I thought this might be the reason for his lack of energy. The autumn evening was cool. It was drizzling.

Riley had been living at Palmer Lodge for two weeks and four days.

"Please go back to the hostel, Riley," I pleaded. "If you get wet and cold, your cough will get worse."

He said that he would. "I'm just taking a walk, to clear my head," he added.

"Isn't it about time for your evening meal, son? Do you know what's for dinner?"

"Re-soles," he said. Riley always referred to rissoles as re-soles.

"That's one of your favourites, Ril. Why don't you go home and have your dinner while it's hot."

"Yeah, yeah, Mum. Whatever."

"I love you, Ril," I said at the end of the call. I never spoke to my son again.

Following the call, Kevin and I went to the city to buy a gift for a wedding that we were to attend soon. When we arrived home around 9.00pm, there was a muddled message on the answering machine from a distressed female. The message concerned Riley and she mumbled a contact phone number.

"Rewind it, Kevin," I implored him. "I can't understand her. Play it again."

"3804…something…71...what? I can't make the numbers out. She's saying it too fast. Can I slow this thing down?" He prodded all the buttons.

"Play it again, Kevin."

"Let's try phoning combinations of the numbers," he suggested.

We played the message over and over. We phoned every possible combination of the mumbled numbers, but got no answers. The first four digits, which we could clearly decipher, were for government and public service offices in the city, but when adding combinations of the other numbers, we only succeeded in connecting to recorded messages, as it was after business hours. We were baffled. Such phone messages had become commonplace in our household over the years as the confusion and mayhem of Riley's life escalated.

I had, as a result, developed an anxiety about the phone. It was so often the bearer of bad news and represented issues that I did not want to face. Whenever it rang, I tensed, my mouth dried, and my clammy hands trembled. If I answered it, I had difficulty hearing the opening greeting because my hearing was distorted by blood pumping hard through my ears. I gulped for breath.

If it was a friendly call, I still took moments to compose myself and respond in an appropriate manner. I often got messages wrong because I was flustered and couldn't comprehend what was being said. If the call concerned Riley, my mind automatically switched to survival tactics: *Take deep breaths. Stay calm. Get details. Which hospital? We're on our way.*

When Kevin took the call, my physical and emotional distress was even worse. I watched his body language for a sign, painful seconds passing as he listened to the caller. Even the slightest tensing of his jaw told me it was bad news. If he relaxed, I almost cried with relief.

And phone calls that came outside reasonable hours were especially traumatic, all the more so when they did not concern

Riley. I had to restrain myself from shouting at late callers, 'Why are you calling so late? Don't you realise how distressing late-night phone calls are in our household?'

With the passing of years after Riley's death, these responses have lessened, but they have never really left me. I would gladly remove the phone from my home to exorcise the memories that it evokes. And these irrationalities probably explain why I am reluctant to use a mobile phone.

Although we were concerned about this indecipherable message on the answering machine, we went to bed with the thought that we would contact Riley the following day.

When I woke early on Saturday morning 17th May 1997, I was aware that the rain had continued throughout the cool night, and my waking thought was that I hoped Riley had not been out in it, making his cough worse. We were reading the newspapers and having a cup of tea when I heard a knock at the front door. Kevin went to the door, and, when I heard his anguished cry, I knew instinctively that Riley was dead. At 7.45am, two police officers came to our home to tell us that Riley had died during the night by hanging himself from playground equipment in the park near his hostel accommodation. He had been out in the cool, wet night.

The two police officers were kind and although my recollections of that fateful morning are mostly surreal fragments of memory, I remember that they were sensitive to our distress. While Kevin and I dressed to go with them to the John Tonge Centre to identify Riley, they offered several times to make us tea or coffee. And one of them followed me through the house as I locked doors.

"What about that one?" he asked. "You didn't lock it."

"It's okay," I assured him. "There's an outside door that is locked."

"Let's lock it, eh? Best not to take any chances."

His concern comforted me.

The rain that had dampened my son during his last night had ceased as we drove to the mortuary, but low dark clouds followed us. The officers in the front of the car spoke quietly with each other and left Kevin and me to our private sorrow in the back. The journey unfolded like a disjointed dream. Outside the car, a *tableau vivant* met my gaze, while inside the car two incidents became embedded in my consciousness.

I heard a voice on the police radio ask our carers to attend another matter. "Sorry, we won't be available for a few hours. We have the parents of a sudden death in the car," he responded.

A sudden death? Was he speaking about Riley? The words seared into my brain. Was this what my beloved son had become? Riley was my corporeal son of twenty-six years and the words stung me. His life was diminished by three inanimate words of police jargon.

Then I became agitated and spoke aloud of my fear that his death had not been 'sudden' enough to spare him pain. Enduring emotional pain had driven him to this moment, but was Riley's last earthly sensation physical suffering? I was tormented.

"I wouldn't think so," said the younger officer. "When people do this sort of thing, they usually have a fair bit of drink on board. You know, a few drinks for courage."

The older officer shot a glare at his colleague. "I can't believe you said that," he snarled through clenched teeth. Silence fell over the four of us as we each pondered our regrets.

Weeks later, I requested Riley's Post-Mortem Examination Report. The analysis indicated that 'Nil' alcohol was present in his blood and urine at the time of his death. I took the report to the psychiatrist who assisted me with my grief following Riley's death. He assured me that although Riley had hanged himself, he 'had made a good death.' He insisted that Riley had felt no pain. I need to believe him.

When we arrived at the John Tonge Centre, we pulled into an empty parking area that was desolate and grey, a reflection of the dismal skies that wept cold raindrops. Brown autumn leaves skittered around the damp car park at the will of swirling wind gusts. I felt that there was no one else in this bleak world but me and my waiting son.

The police officers took us into a small room that resembled a doctor's waiting room: functional chairs against the walls, and

I think there were some plastic flowers on the corner table with magazines. We declined our escorts' offer of tea once more and then they left us for a short time. When they returned, they told us briefly what to expect when we saw Riley. They hesitantly and nervously explained the physical aftermath of hanging. Then they opened the door to the viewing room.

For the fourth time in my life, a glass window separated me from my son. But I did not see the person that the officers had described. I saw my son. He was on a gurney, naked, but covered to his neck by a small sheet. His knees were bent. "His knees are bent! Why are his knees bent?" I was sobbing. I looked at the officers, but they were shaking their heads, mumbling, and stepping back, away from me. No answer. Then I saw the tattoo. Because Riley's knees were bent, they formed an arch that lifted the sheet, exposing a tattooed skull on the outside of his left calf. I knew he had other tattoos, but I didn't know about this one. He had kept it secret because he knew I didn't approve. And his hair was wet. Had someone washed him, or was his hair still wet from last night's rain? My beloved son's hair. Blond. Curly. Wet. I clawed at the glass window separating Riley and myself as I tried to get through to him. My arms were spread in a wide crucifix against the glass as I embraced the window because I desperately wished to embrace my son. My wretchedness filled the room. My sobs were deep gulps that choked me. I will regret for the rest of my life that I didn't ask, didn't insist, that I be allowed to go in to him. To go to the other side of the window. Just to hold him one last time. To feel his cheek against mine, to take his smell with me. In such times of utter grief, precious moments are lost for eternity because one's mind is almost demented with sorrow and a sense that this is not really happening. 'Please let me wake up from this nightmare. Please don't let it be true.'

On the homeward journey, as we drove along the South-East Freeway, the surname of the young officer in the front seat came into my mind. I interrupted my soft weeping. "Micawber. That's an unusual name. I've never heard of a real person with that name. I only know of Micawber as a character in a Dickens' novel." He swivelled in his seat to look at me, bewilderment on his face. He said nothing.

I didn't know if he was intrigued by my literary disclosure or if he was nonplussed that a mother so newly grieved could make such an incidental aside. I resumed my quiet crying, watching the gentle rain form rivulets that trickled down the misted car window.

How had we come to this point? What had happened during Riley's twenty-six years of life that made him want to die? How was it that although I was devastated by his death, I was not surprised? Over the last decade of his intense mental dysfunction, I gradually accepted the inevitably of his death, but I convinced myself that it would happen in the future, and the future is not today, not just now. I appeased my fears with the hope that the future would never actually arrive. But it had.

In the last two weeks of Riley's life, he was unusually calm and appeared to be at peace with himself. He seemed contented. There were no delusions, no expressions of rage, and the glares and huffing and puffing through clenched teeth gave way to composure. He was happy to stand in the kitchen as I prepared meals and chat. He was companionable. He was often in my way at the kitchen bench, but I cherished these moments so much that I worked around him. He knew he was in the way. "I'll do my snake trick, Mum, and hiss off."

"No, Ril. It's okay. I can manage." I knew that these rare moments of communication and quietude were precious, but, sadly, I didn't realise then just how meaningful they would soon become. Although Riley always had periodic times of rationality and pleasantness, this was different. Serenity is a word that I had never associated with Riley in the past, but he had a tranquillity about him that was unfamiliar and puzzled me. I paused several times to ask myself if this seemingly normal person was the same son who could be out of touch with reality, impulsively illogical, and belligerent. At the time, the thought went through my mind that at last this might signal a turning point in his health and that in some way he was overcoming his difficulties and a recovery might be possible. I allowed myself this tentative, rare moment of hope.

After his death, however, I realised that he must have resolved that his time had finally come, and that for those two weeks he was at peace with his decision.

It was not unusual for Riley to check into a motel and attempt suicide. But he always phoned either us, his psychiatrist, the police, or the ambulance to come to his rescue, and it was this habit that lulled us into the belief that he would always seek help and be saved. Although we were warned that one of these attempts could accidentally lead to his death, his final act was not an accident. He made sure no passer-by could intervene and nor could he make that vital phone call. He had finally determined that he no longer wished to endure the emotional pain that plagued his life, and he sought relief in death. He decided his own final decide. Although we are grief-stricken, we respect and understand his decision.

In the weeks that followed Riley's death, Kevin and I were taken by the police, at my request, to Gilmour Park. It was explained to me by the psychiatrist who counselled me that in general, men are satisfied with knowledge of the big picture, but women mostly need to know every little detail that goes into that picture. Accordingly, I asked the policeman who attended Riley's death to tell me all those details. I needed to know. And I needed to be assured that Riley had been treated with dignity.

We met the officer at the Redcliffe Police Station. He was quiet, and he seemed to me to be distressed. In a faltering voice, he explained the unfolding of events on that morning. Kevin and I listened attentively, asking some questions. Then he said, "Riley was found hanging from the second rung of the climbing frame in a kneeling position." A kneeling position? Was this why his knees were bent when we identified him at John Tonge?

"He was kneeling?" I asked the officer for confirmation. "You mean that he could have stood up if he wanted to? He could have put his feet on the ground?"

"Yes. But he didn't."

Kevin and I collapsed into each other's arms, with inconsolable sobs. I remember the wetness of our tears. "He meant to do it! He really meant to do it! He could have stopped, he could have saved himself, but he didn't!" Which one of us said this? I don't know. Perhaps we both did. It was gut wrenching to know that Riley was so determined, yet at the same time, consoling to know that this was what he wanted.

The officer then drove us to Gilmour Park. It's funny how trivial things stick in one's mind and become memories that are so readily recalled. I remember that the officer had to remove rubbish from the car to clear the seats for us.

When we arrived, once again the officer recounted and demonstrated aspects from that morning, then he left Kevin and me alone to reflect on our son's life and mourn his death. This was when we found the white wooden cross with Riley's name on it, under a young jacaranda tree. We were comforting and consoling each other when another question occurred to me. I looked back for the officer and saw him leaning against the police car, arms folded across his chest, head down, crying. I went to him and put my hand on his arm.

"I could be you," he said, sniffing back his distress. "You and your husband. It could be me and my wife. Grieving and crying like you. Our daughter tried to kill herself last week. She cut her wrists. God, it's a nightmare. What can we do to keep our kids safe? Alive? What are parents supposed to do?"

"Go home and hug her and love her," I told him.

We make an early-morning pilgrimage to Gilmour Park on the 17th May every year and it is a difficult journey. Flocks of birds are always twittering busily in the old gum tree to greet the break of day when we arrive at 6.30am. Cars pass, taking drivers to dawn destinations, while pedestrians stride out their sunrise walk, or return from the corner shop with milk and newspapers. In my moments of deepest grief, I am acutely aware that nature does not pause for sorrow. Nor does the hum of life diminish.

Because of his love for Tugun, on the rare occasions when Riley had cause to celebrate, such as when he had completed a stint of community service or paid off a fine, he would ask us to take him to Tugun where he indulged in a meat pie and pineapple tart from the local bakery. When eating the pie, he would lick each finger meticulously to savour every last drop of pie gravy. Then, with us, he would climb the Elephant Rock lookout and shout into the wind, "I'm free! I'm free!" His head was thrown back with his face to the blue sky, arms reaching out in exaltation in the air. The sound of the pounding surf and the cawing of gulls that soared above him on wafts of wind accompanied his joyous chorus.

So each year on the anniversary of his death, Kevin and I go to Tugun. We have a meat pie and a pineapple tart, and then we climb the Elephant Rock lookout. Together we stand facing into the wind. "You're free, Riley! You are free, son!" we shout at the top of our lungs, in memory of our Riley. All we ever wanted was for Riley to be free: free of bullies, free of a judgemental society that excluded the mentally ill, free to participate at his level and without prejudice within his community, and most of all, free of his illness.

Obviously, Tugun equated to a sense of peace and well being for Riley and because of this, we scattered his ashes there, in the dunes and in the sea. We hope that by making Tugun his final resting place, we have given him freedom and eternal peace in a place that he loved.

Chapter 18

Blurb from the Stepping Stone Clubhouse brochure states:

> *Stepping Stone is a prevocational rehabilitation day program for people with psychiatric disabilities who are striving to become more productive, self-sufficient members of our community. Stepping Stone is a private, not for profit organisation established on the 5th of September 1994 by the Schizophrenia Fellowship of South Queensland, Inc.*

Members, as participants in Stepping Stone are called, work side by side with staff in a Work Ordered Day (WOD) with an aim to achieve Transitional Employment (TE), Supported Employment (SE), or Independent Employment (IE). Stepping Stone also provides a Supported Education program for members who may require specific skills, or for those members who wish to improve their education.

Members also welcome the opportunity to speak in public forums about mental health issues and the role Stepping Stone has in helping them to achieve their goals.

Melanie Sennett, Director of Stepping Stone adds that the Clubhouse has an holistic, rather than a medical philosophy where people are recognised as people, not patients. Stepping Stone believes that everyone has a contribution to make, based on a strength approach, and that every individual has skills, talents, and abilities to offer. Members are involved in every aspect of running the Clubhouse and they hold positions on the management committee. Stepping Stone Clubhouse also offers a social recreational program on evenings and weekends and is open every public holiday. This is extremely important because many of their members do not have family with whom to spend the holidays.

What impressed me about the staff at Stepping Stone was the non-judgemental, unconditional support provided for members. A slogan I heard repeatedly said, 'Once a member, always a member.'

A quote by Propst, Beard and Malamud in the Stepping Stone brochure best captures their guiding principles:

Work, and the potential to aspire to gainful employment is a deeply regenerative and reintegrating force in the life of every human being.

Two words encapsulate what Stepping Stone offers its members: Dignity and Hope.

Riley was an inaugural member of Brisbane's Stepping Stone Clubhouse and his time as a member of the organisation was the one positive and promising period in his life. He was an active member of Stepping Stone for the last two-and-a-half years of his life, and this wonderful group of people provided some purpose and daily structure for him.

He learnt computer skills at Stepping Stone, and took pleasure in dazzling me with technical jargon. He took his turn at preparing the lunchtime meal for members each day, and was proud of his involvement in the organisation of their first national conference.

He kept a running diary of the preparations he was involved in for the conference, and gave an address to the plenary session. This is an extract from his notes in preparation for his speech:

> *Good Morning, my name is Riley Brasch. I am a member of Stepping Stone in the good old town of Brisbane. I am going to speak to you about the history and development of Stepping Stone. In Brisbane, Stepping Stone clubhouse has already firmly established its roots, and to many, me especially has become a life saver. It is the best rehabilitation I have come accross since my illness 7 years ago. Prior to this programme I have tryed just about every thing, but Stepping Stone has proven to be the most successful. At the clubhouse we have a great thing called the work ordered day. This includes Staff and members working side by side to get the work for the day done.*

He also participated in the official function to open Stepping Stone where he was selected to be host to Peter Beattie, the Premier of Queensland, and together they cut the ribbon to declare Stepping Stone officially open. A photo of this, along with a letter of appreciation for his contribution to the national conference, is framed and displayed with pride in our home.

Apart from our daughter, a member of Stepping Stone was the

only other speaker at Riley's funeral.

On the day of Riley's funeral, I didn't cry. Coby was giving the eulogy and I knew how difficult this was for her. I willed myself to be strong and composed because I knew that if I broke down, Coby's task would be impossible. My eyes didn't leave Coby as she spoke from the lectern and I tried with every fibre in my body to transmit to her my love and my admiration for her courage. She was magnificent. Behind me, I could hear someone sobbing.

I remember the beautiful floral arrangement of white lithianthus and orange tulips that covered Riley's coffin. I had asked the florist to make certain that his flowers were special, and they were. And our home was so inundated with floral tributes that they filled every flat surface in the lounge room, dining room, and spilled over to the patio and outside veranda.

I look back on Riley's funeral, and it feels as if I wasn't there, someone else was, and I was just watching from afar. Even now, I ask Kevin questions about Riley's funeral because there is so much that I can't remember.

But I do remember hundreds of people at Riley's funeral, though I can't recall the words of comfort they tried to convey to me. I can only remember kind faces with mouths that opened and closed but I heard no words. A silent movie replays in my memory.

I remember seeing my much-loved uncle at the back of the crowd, but he didn't speak to me. My aunt told me later that he could not find adequate words to do my sorrow justice.

And I remember all the people at my home after the funeral, but I can't remember how I interacted with our guests. I have to read the attendance book that records more than three hundred names of people who came to Riley's funeral to know who was there. Among these names are many of Riley's Stepping Stone friends.

His good friend and mentor from Stepping Stone, Warren Sparrow, read this letter of appreciation at Riley's funeral:

> *Dear Kevin, Tilly and Jacoba*
>
> *We received news of Riley's death with great sadness. Riley was a valued member of Stepping Stone and he will be missed by many people for many years.*
>
> *Riley was one of the first people to join our program.*

He was here the very first day we opened and is one of only three that stuck with it to this day. Riley has made a very big impact on our community.

I think we saw a side of Riley that very few people saw. At Stepping Stone, he always had a smile on his face, he came ready and willing to work all day, almost every day. He made friends easily, and made sure new members to the Clubhouse felt welcomed and were not alone. In the two and half years he spent with us, he gave over 300 tours and explained what we do to over 1500 people. He took pride in his contribution, he was very good at it, and he was always willing to do more.

Riley spoke to me often about his family. I know he had a tumultuous life, but he loved and admired you both, as well as his sister. When he spoke about you, it was always with an unerring sense of pride. He was distressed at times over the grief he caused, but he was always thinking of ways to make amends. That usually was putting his head down and proving himself in one way or another.

Please accept my deepest sympathy for your loss. I personally shall miss Riley terribly. Regardless of my role as Director of Stepping Stone, I have always considered Riley to be a friend. I admired his courage and determination, as well as his sense of humour, in a life filled with adversity.

I hope with all my heart his struggle is now at an end. I know he will now be resting. And, I know he shall be looking down upon his family that he loved so much, to take care of them.

On behalf of all of the members, staff and Committee of Management please accept our most sincere condolences.

Yours truly

Warren Sparrow MSW

Chapter 19

I am unable to use the phrase 'committed suicide' and always flinch when I hear it used in other forums. 'Committed' implies the transmission of some wrongdoing, as in 'committed a sin' or 'committed a crime.' People like Riley who take their lives mostly are seeking release from the emotional and physical torment they have endured in life. They have committed no wrong, except for wishing to be normal and accepted, to be treated compassionately, to have some dignity, and most of all, to be free of illness. Nonetheless, a wrong *is* committed when someone completes suicide, but it is committed by those who have failed to provide the understanding and support this minority so desperately seeks.

Prior to Riley's death, I was a competent cook. The last meal that I cooked for Riley had him proclaiming: "Who is all this food for Mum? It's just you and Dad and me. Not the whole damn street! But, you've done it again. Great tucker! You've excelled yourself!" And he always gave me a mark for presentation, or *preee-zen-tation* as he liked to say in an exaggerated American accent: 'Preee-zen-tation, fifteen out of ten!' was his usual score for me especially when I made his favourite party food, Stuffed *Up* Eggs, a Rileyism, which is what we still call Stuffed Eggs.

But after his death, I couldn't think what to cook. Nor could I manage the basic preparation of an easy meal. And I couldn't follow a simple recipe. I'd stare at the words for ages, repeating the straightforward instructions over and over, and not have a clue how to make a start. Mostly, I stopped cooking: frozen meals and take-aways became our staple diet. For months, it was only through the kindness of a few friends that Kevin and I ate anything other than basic fare. I even took myself off to cooking classes, hoping not only to regain the confidence of my previous ability, but that through this domestic procedure, I would learn how to live a normal life again. Even now, after more than seven years, I still have a problem with cooking. I think this is because I subconsciously associate cooking with nurturing Riley, and this is no longer possible.

My friend Ruby, whose son died in a motor vehicle accident many years before we lost Riley, took the opposite approach to cooking after Graham died. When I called to see her in the days, weeks, months following Graham's death, I'd find her in the kitchen cooking batches of biscuits or icing cakes. "What on earth are you doing, Ruby? Do you really need to be doing this?"

"It's the only way I can cope, Tilly. When I'm cooking, I feel normal," she replied.

Following Riley's death, I preferred to be a social dropout because of my lack of confidence. Kevin's involvement in sport and his corporate positions mean that we are invited to many social functions. Prior to Riley's death, I was committed to supporting Kevin and happy to be a sociable person. When an invitation arrived I'd ask, "Does it include dinner?"

"Yes, they'll feed us," Kevin affirmed.

"Good. I do enjoy a meal that I don't have to cook. Now, what will I wear?" was my standard response.

But now, I prefer to stay at home. "Do I have to go? Do you really need me there?" I ask.

What I dread most about going into social situations is the inevitable question, "Do you have any children?" I still haven't worked out a suitable answer. I *do* have two children, and when I am asked about them, what should I say about Riley that doesn't make people feel uncomfortable? Death, and more particularly suicide, are not subjects that make for easy social interaction. But I will not gloss over, nor deny Riley's life. The easy way out for me is to avoid situations where such questions might be asked.

Tasks which I previously undertook without a second thought became a nightmare of anticipation for me after Riley's death. I began to experience panic attacks. My job required me to speak in an advisory capacity to people throughout the day, mostly just one person at a time, or often a small group, and sometimes, several hundred people. I used to love it and did it well. But, after Riley's death, I was tongue-tied. I stammered and stuttered and constantly lost my train of thought. I dreaded this aspect of my job and I was often embarrassed by my poor performance.

In the months following Riley's death, I had another university exam to sit. Before Riley died, I took university exams in my stride, even relishing the challenges. 'Let me at it!' was my usual approach. But now, anxiety entered the exam room with me.

"There are ten essay topics on the paper," the invigilator announced. "You are required to select three topics from the ten for your written essays. You may commence now."

At first, I couldn't read the paper. The words blurred before my eyes. I couldn't breath. I thought I was having an asthma attack. My hand shook making it difficult to hold my pen to make notes. Three essays, I thought as I perused the paper, squinting to decipher the words. What are my options? Not much of a choice. Bloody hell, there's nothing here that I've prepared for! With blurred vision, gasping for breath, and trembling hand, I wrote three essays.

When the exam was over, we sat waiting for the supervisors to collect our scripts. I looked over at the paper written by the student sitting next to me. "Where did you get those topics from?" I asked her.

"Here," she said, turning the question paper over. Five topics were on the front of the paper, and five were on the back. But it hadn't occurred to me to turn the paper over. I had read only five topics from the front of the paper. Instead of a choice of three essays out of ten, I had limited myself to three out of five. The topics that I had studied for were on the back of the question paper.

For many years after Riley died, I could not stop myself from sorting all days, dates, events, and recollections, irrespective of whether they related to Riley or not, into BR — Before Riley (died), and AR — After Riley. And there was only one day of the week that was okay for me: Thursday. Every other day of the week had a specific memory of something to do with Riley's death, but Thursdays were 'safe'. My world fell into two distinct eras, one when I physically had a son and the other where I only have intangible memories.

Even now, more than seven years after losing him, at the end of each day when I take stock of how the day has turned out, I think of Riley. Whether the day has been good or otherwise, whether I am happy or not so pleased with things, I am aware of Riley's absence.

I wonder how my day would have involved him, but I know that he isn't here. He is like a shadow that is just out of my vision. I can sense him, but I know he isn't with me. He will never be with me again.

For months after Riley died, I awoke most mornings and thought, 'It was only a horrible dream. But I'm awake now. It will be alright now.' But the spectres that came to me in the night were not the instruments of my torture. The torturous nightmare was the reality of my waking hours. And even though I craved the restorative power of sleep, I dreaded the dark hours when I lay awake with my tormented thoughts.

We replaced many years of heartache, turmoil, mental anguish, and a sense of total failure with profound grief. But our grief was not only about his death. It was also about his life.

As I try to think through my emotions, I question how my experience of motherhood moved from the elation and joy of holding my newborn baby after birth, soaking up his smell, and the softness of his warm skin, to seeing that same child in a mortuary, and later kissing his cold, rigid body goodbye in his coffin. The profundity of this emotion can never be explained, understood, or imagined, but only felt, in a way that transcends the deepest sorrow.

Literature about suicide and bereavement counsellors explains that grief is an individual process. There is no right or wrong way to express one's grief. In general, males grieve differently from females, and each person grieves differently from others. But it is important to be allowed to grieve, to rage with anger at the senselessness of a lost life, and to cry bittersweet tears of memory, instead of keeping a stiff upper lip.

In the earlier stages of my grief, I felt disconnected with the world around me. I became mechanical, devoid of joy and laughter. On occasions when I did allow myself to laugh, I would stop suddenly, consumed with guilt that I was laughing and my son was dead. Laughter seemed profane to me.

In my grief, the love and kindness of others sustained me in my darkest moments, but one remark still haunts me. This particular sympathiser said to me as we stood in the supermarket aisle, "I'm so sorry about your loss. It must be awful for you. But he *was* flawed, wasn't he? I guess it's not like you've lost a normal child, is it? Perhaps it was for the best."

Was this meant to console me? I needed counselling before I could accept that the remark was merely thoughtless and not meant to hurt me.

But a kind friend asked me, two years after Riley's death: "Where are you at with your grieving, Tilly?" This question acknowledged that I could still be grieving and it warmed my heart. And she listened quietly while I told her about the stages of my ongoing grief. I treasured my friend's sensitivity, but it was a rare experience. More commonly I am asked: "How are you going, Til? Back to normal?" And even before I have a chance to respond, the inquirer quickly moves to another topic of conversation to circumvent the uncomfortable possibility that I might say, "Well, actually, I'm still grieving. No, I'm not 'back to normal', whatever that might mean."

There is an expectation in our society that people who have lost a loved one should soon 'come to terms' with the death and 'accept' their loss. This may be a reasonable expectation when the lost loved one is elderly and has lived a full and happy life. Such a death is a normal and natural rite of passage.

But how can I 'come to terms' with, and 'accept' that my young son chose to die so tragically after a short and difficult life? My experience has made it clear to me that our culture is afraid of death, and quickly becomes impatient with prolonged grieving. It's okay, allowable, to grieve for two or three weeks, but after that, it is expected that the grief-stricken person should 'get on with it', and if they don't, then they are deemed to be indulging in morbidity, or perhaps their loss has unbalanced the mind.

Recently, a young Greek friend lost her husband after a long battle with cancer. I attended his funeral, and Sophia told me that in nine days time, then forty days, she would participate in other rituals with family and friends to honour her husband's memory. There will be other shared, ritualistic milestones throughout the first year as well. Her loss will continue to be recognised and she will be supported in her grief.

This shared and supportive attitude for an extended grieving period is not unusual among other cultures. These cultures seem to understand and recognise that a person suffering a loss should not go through the processes alone, and that grief is a prolonged emotion, not something that can be quickly resolved.

In the Vietnamese culture, there is an intense series of rituals and memorial services during the first year of loss which:

"…forced the family to burden others with their sorrow so that they could grieve fully. Each successive memorial was held a little less frequently as the family became more able to resume some form of ordinary routine….The socially prescribed rituals from the time of death until the end of the mourning period are designed to provide a structure for the grief process."

This extended grieving process, shared by family, friends, and the community is also observed in Hindu and Muslim religions.

Contrast this with the attitude of my work-place supervisor, two weeks after a colleague's young son was killed in a motor vehicle accident. "Where's Ruby? Is she back yet?" he barked.

"No," I replied. "It's only been two weeks since Graham died," I reminded him.

"I know that! How much time does she want to weep and wail? If she wants to keep her job, she'd better be at her desk on Monday." His reaction appalled me.

The truth is that these attitudes and expectations only serve to make the grieving process more difficult. It is more than seven years now since we lost Riley and I still grieve, but because of society's demands, because of the expectation of stoic silence and a stiff upper lip, I am forced to do it in private. My public persona is one of being happy and getting on with my life, and in general, this is true. But I still have many painful, reflective moments when quiet tears flow. Physically, my son was part of my life for almost twenty-six years. I can still hear his voice and his husky chuckle, and see his crooked grin: eternal love for ephemeral flesh.

The fact that Riley died doesn't make him any less an important part of my life, a son with whom I shared so many experiences which continue to shape my life and are part of the composite person that I am. But I don't want to speak about his death — I want to speak about his life and how it entwined with mine. I want to speak of the times that are happy memories, the times that put a smile on my face then, and still do now. But most people go quiet when I mention Riley's name and I feel as if I have committed a social gaffe.

I cut an article from *The Courier-Mail* after Riley's death that expresses my thoughts:

> *...it helps to talk, not so much about the suicide but about the person, your child, because they mean so much to you....The value and meaning of my son's life has not been cancelled out by his death.*

In the weeks that followed Riley's death, when we were being inundated with many forms of sympathy, I unconsciously sorted the people I knew into three groups:

The first are those who you know care, and they do all in their power to show their love and support. How would I have survived without them?

The second are those who are not necessarily close friends, but gave solace when they made unexpected contact, went out of their way, to visit, phone, or write. This sort of contact gave me an inner warmth and deep sense of comfort.

Then there is the third group, people who I know well and see regularly. But not a word, not even a card on which they only had to sign their name. I know they do not mean me harm, but I am bewildered by their silence.

On the first day that I returned to work after Riley's death, one of my colleagues saw me, opened his arms wide, and said, "You need a hug." How comforting this simple, kind gesture was in comparison with another colleague who looked startled when he saw me, and after spluttering incoherently for a few seconds, walked away. Not a word. Unfortunately, I often encountered silence. It seemed to me that many people skirted around me and avoided me, but I was deeply touched and comforted by those who took the trouble to make contact with me. A hug, a kind word, or taking the time to talk and listen, can be so comforting and healing.

I acknowledge that most people think they are being considerate by not mentioning my lost son because they think they are protecting me from becoming upset. However, being upset is part of the grieving process, a vital cathartic process, just as laughing is part of being happy, and we all enjoy sharing in happy times. Sometimes I feel a great need to express my feelings and thoughts, but grief is an extremely lonely and isolating emotion. It seems that grief has to be adjusted to accommodate those who have not suffered the loss, in case they are made to feel uncomfortable.

In *Much Ado About Nothing*, Shakespeare wrote: '*Every one can master a grief, But he that has it.*'

If I had to explain the grieving process to someone who has not experienced the loss of a child, I would use the analogy of recovering from serious surgery. At first, the wound is open and raw, and therefore obvious to others. Initially, there is support, understanding and sympathy for the enormous pain and suffering that is being endured. But as the open wound appears to outwardly heal, so too do people grow weary of continuing to hear ongoing details. However, for the sufferer, what remains is a deep ache and a scar that is always sensitive. Allowances have to be made to incorporate the ache and scar into daily life, and certain conditions or circumstances bring on a return of discomfort. The wound may even flare every now and then. The scarred person is constantly reminded of the original wound in a painful manner. And even though the scar may fade with the years, it is a lifetime legacy, always there, always tender, always in need of gentle treatment.

Postscript

Writing this account has been a difficult journey through memories that, at best, are painful, and, at worst, are locked away in a corner of my mind because they are too distressing to consciously acknowledge to myself, let alone to a reader. Therefore, this will always be an incomplete record of Riley's life.

But at the most unlikely moment, or in some insignificant situation, something — a sight, a smell, a sound, a sensation — will trigger a long-forgotten memory and so much pain comes flooding back. Sometimes I dream of Riley and feel cheated when I wake up and realise that he wasn't really with me. It was only a dream. Gone. Dreams and memories are all that I have of him now.

Apart from loving Riley and treasuring his memory, I am indebted to him for the greater dimensions of understanding and compassion that I now possess and my heightened awareness of how precious and transient a life can be. Sometimes when I think back on his life, I have to ask myself, did he really exist? He seems to have come in and out of my life so swiftly, for just a brief moment in my lifetime. I think of him as a gentle breeze that blew softly on my skin, and then was gone. No more.

I want to make this record of his life so that those who read it might have an insight into his difficulties and know that although he was troubled, he was kind, brave, and funny.

It is also important to me that I record Riley's short and difficult life because he will have no children or grandchildren to carry forward the family stories of what their father or grandfather did or said. This record is his final history. Unless his life is written down in this manner, all knowledge of him will die with his immediate family.

Riley became an uncle after he died and because he was so gentle, generous, and loving, I know that he would have loved Madison and Darcy unconditionally, with all his heart. I hope that by reading this, his nieces might understand the uncle they never knew, and be as proud of him as I am. I hope that they can hold him in a special place in their memories.

People have asked me how I survived the years of Riley's illness, and I ask, 'What were my options?' Indeed, what are the realistic options? I could have deadened my daily sorrow with alcohol or pills. I could have displayed our constant turbulence like a black armband. Or I could have chosen to sink into depression. But I resolved to get on with my life as positively as I could. I owe this much to Riley, who, with his flawed logic and tragic reasoning, believed that he was not only setting himself free of his misery by ending his life, but that he was also freeing his family from the constant trauma that his illness brought into our every day. And now that he is no longer with us, we should not fritter away this new life that follows my son's last tragic sacrifice for those he loved.

Nevertheless, he may have freed us from the turmoil that was our former life, but this does not mean that our lives are free from ongoing anguish, or that we love him less with the passing of the years. Not a day, and sometimes not an hour passes that I don't think of Riley. My love didn't die with him and he will always be my son. Although I don't believe in an afterlife, I do know that Riley is no longer suffering earthly torment, and I know that he did not want me to suffer. He often said to me of his illness, "This is not your fault, Mum," and I know that is true, yet I still feel deep in my heart that I should have been able to save him, to 'catch' him. But I didn't. I couldn't. That is a fact that I cannot alter, and the best that I can do now for Riley is to live my life to the fullest. He would wish me no less. Kevin expressed it in this poem he wrote for Riley's funeral:

Grieve not for me,
For now I am free.
My world is not your world,
And so it must be.
With this step I have taken,
All my troubles will cease.
So Mum, Dad, and Coby
Please share in my peace.

Riley's Medical Time Line

1984/86	Private psychiatric out-patient
1986/1993	Intermittent public psychiatric in-patient; Placement in hostels; Periods of independent living
23/7/93 - 26/2/97	Private hospital in-patient; Occasional 'transitional' accommodation at good hostel
26/2/97 - 21/3/97	Intermittent public psychiatric in-patient
21/3/97 - 28/4/97	Public hospital placement in good hostel accommodation; Two days as public psychiatric in-patient
28/4/97 - 16/5/97	Palmer Lodge

References

Chapter 1

For information on dysmaturity, or intrauterine growth retardation, see *General Health Encyclopaedia* at: http://www.healthcentral. com/mhc/top/001500.cfm

For information on postmaturity, see *The Merck Manual – Second Home Edition*, at: http://www.msd-australia.com.au/mrkshared/mmanual_home2/sec23/ch264/ch264d.jsp

For information on placental insufficiency, see Professor M.G. Elder of London's Hammersmith Hospital, Royal Postgraduate School at: http://www.child.org.uk/html/malta.php/factsheets/72/

Chapter 2

For information on bone age tests, see: http://www.drhull.com/EncyMaster/B/bone_age.html

Chapter 4

Dare to care: SANE Mental Health Report 2004.

Royal Australian and New Zealand College of Psychiatrists (Queensland), in 'Mental Illness and violence plague homeless people' (8). *The Courier-Mail*, Wednesday March 2, 2005.

Sundin, Dr Josey. *The Courier-Mail*, Wednesday March 2, 2005. 'Mental illness and violence plague homeless people' (8). Jeff Sommerfeld.

Walker, Judge Frank, President Schizophrenia Fellowship of NSW Inc, *Symposium 2003: Out of the Darkness and into the Light*, at: http://www.sfnsw.org.au/publications/Frank%20Walker%2003.pdf

Chapter 6

John, Elton. *'Candle in the Wind'*, on *Goodbye Yellow Brick Road, 1997.*

Chapter 13

Wilkie, Dr William, *The Courier-Mail*, Monday 2 February 2004. 'Shock therapy use tops other states' (3). Leanne Edmistone, Health Reporter.

Queensland Government, Department of Justice and Attorney General. *Guardianship*, at: http://www.justice.qld.gov.au/guardian/home.htm

The Courier-Mail, Monday 2 February 2004. 'Shock therapy use tops other states' (3). Leanne Edmistone, Health Reporter.

Chapter 15

'Mental hostels squalor exposed'. *The Courier-Mail*, Thursday December 23, 2004 (1). Margaret Wenham.

Chapter 16

Beattie, Peter, MLA. Correspondence, 18 July 2000.

Brasch, Jacoba. 'The Human Rights of Mental Illness: Involuntary Commitment and Treatment in Australia and USA'. 2nd USA Pacific Law Conference, New York, 21-27 April 2003.

Groom, Dr Grace and Professor Ian Hickie. *A Review of Mental Health Services in Australia – 2003: 'Out of Hospital, Out of Mind!'*, at: http://www.mhca.com.au/Public/PoliciesDocumentation/OutHospitalOutofMind_FinalReport.pdf

'Hospital closes mental health beds'. *The Courier-Mail*, Wednesday January 19, 2005 (3). Jeff Sommerfeld, Health Reporter.

Moore, Clover. *Mental Health Services: Matter of Public Importance*. 12 November 2003, at: http://www.clovermoore.com/speeches/2003/031112-1.htm

Nordern, Father Peter, Victoria's Catholic Social Service Secretariat. Quoted in Peter Boyle, *Governments prepare to bury mental health report*, at: http://www.greenleft.org.au/back/1993/121/121p3.htm

Queensland Alliance of Mental Illness and Psychiatric Disability Groups Inc, in 'Hospital closes mental health beds'. *The Courier-Mail*, Wednesday January 19, 2005 (3). Jeff Sommerfeld, Health Reporter.

Queensland Government 2004-05 Budget snapshot, at: http://www.budget.qld.gov.au/budget-papers/budget-snapshot.html

Queensland Government 2003-04 Budget snapshot, at http://www.treasury.qld.gov.au/budget/2003/

Royal Australian and New Zealand College of Psychiatrists (Queensland), in 'Mental illness and violence plague homeless people ' (8). *The Courier-Mail*, Wednesday March 2, 2005.

Chapter 19

Dieu-Hien T. Hoang, RN. *Death Rituals in Vietnamese Society*, (3) at: http://www.ethnomed.org/ethnomed/cultures/vietnamese/viet_death.html

Emergency and Support Contacts

In an emergency, call 000.

Consult Community Help (Health & Help) in front section of the *White Pages* for mental health associations in your region.

To find out what mental health services are available in your area, call **Lifeline's Just Ask information line on 1300 131 114.**

SANE Mental Illness Helpline (Mon to Fri, 9.00am - 5.00pm EST) Freecall 1800 688 382.

SOSBSA - Survivors of Suicide Bereavement Support Association (Grief counseling for the bereaved by suicide & counseling for those at risk of suicide): 1300 767 022.

Stepping Stone Clubhouse, Coorparoo, Qld	(07) 3847 1085
Bridges Clubhouse, Bundaberg, Qld	(07) 4154 2300
Canefields Clubhouse, Beenleigh, Qld	(07) 3807 0951
Jacaranda Clubhouse, Ipswich, Qld	(07) 3812 9771
Federation Clubhouse, Southport, Qld	(07) 5591 1750
Toowoomba Clubhouse, Toowoomba, Qld	(074) 632 4688
Billabong Clubhouse, Tamworth, NSW	(02) 6766 9960
Pioneer Clubhouse, Balgowlah, NSW	(02) 9907 9999
Eureka Clubhouse, Moohah, Tas	(03) 6278 9179
Bromham Place Clubhouse, Richmond, Vic	(03) 9427 7377
Diamond Clubhouse, Kilkenny, SA	(08) 8244 5525

ARAFMI (Support for families caring for someone with mental illness)

Qld: (07) 3254 1881
NSW: (02) 9805 1883
NT: (08) 8942 2811
SA: (08) 8221 5166
Tas: (03) 6236 9251
NSW country areas: Toll Free 1800 655 198)
WA: (08) 9228 0577
Vic: (03) 9889 3733

The Compassionate Friends (Support group for bereaved parents)

Qld: (07) 3254 2657
NSW: (02) 9290 2355
Tas: 1800 641 091
Vic: (03) 9888 4944
SA: (08) 8351 0344
WA: 1800 628 118

Mental Health Associations (Information & referral, education & job training, advocacy & personal support, publications & library)

Qld: (07) 3271 5544; 1300 729 686
NSW: (02) 9816 5688; 1800 674 200
Tas: (03) 6230 7711
NT: (08) 8999 4988
Vic: 1300 650 172
ACT: (02) 6207 5111; 13 22 81
WA: 1800 220 400
SA: 13 14 65

White Wreaths Association

For branches throughout Australia, contact: Brisbane, Qld (Head Office) (07) 3219 7279